PENGUIN BOOKS

A PLACE OF MY OWN

Michael Pollan is the author of nine books, including *This Is Your Mind on Plants, How to Change Your Mind, Cooked, Food Rules, In Defense of Food, The Omnivore's Dilemma,* and *The Botany of Desire,* all of which were *New York Times* bestsellers. He is also the author of the audiobook *Caffeine: How Coffee and Tea Created the Modern World.* A longtime contributor to *The New York Times Magazine,* Pollan teaches writing at Harvard University and the University of California, Berkeley. In 2010, *Time* magazine named him one of the one hundred most influential people in the world.

michaelpollan.com

A Place
of My Own

THE ARCHITECTURE OF

DAYDREAMS

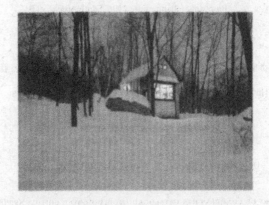

Michael Pollan

PENGUIN BOOKS

PENGUIN BOOKS
Published by the Penguin Group
Penguin Group (USA) Inc., 375 Hudson Street, New York, New York 10014, U.S.A.
Penguin Group (Canada), 90 Eglinton Avenue East, Suite 700, Toronto,
Ontario, Canada M4P 2Y3 (a division of Pearson Penguin Canada Inc.)
Penguin Books Ltd, 80 Strand, London WC2R 0RL, England
Penguin Ireland, 25 St Stephen's Green, Dublin 2, Ireland (a division of Penguin Books Ltd)
Penguin Group (Australia), 250 Camberwell Road, Camberwell,
Victoria 3124, Australia (a division of Pearson Australia Group Pty Ltd)
Penguin Books India Pvt Ltd, 11 Community Centre,
Panchsheel Park, New Delhi – 110 017, India
Penguin Group (NZ), 67 Apollo Drive, Rosedale, North Shore 0632,
New Zealand (a division of Pearson New Zealand Ltd)
Penguin Books (South Africa) (Pty) Ltd, 24 Sturdee Avenue,
Rosebank, Johannesburg 2196, South Africa

Penguin Books Ltd, Registered Offices:
80 Strand, London WC2R 0RL, England

First published in the United States of America by Random House, Inc., 1997
Published by arrangement with Random House, Inc.
This edition with a new preface published in Penguin Books 2008

Printed in the United States of America

23RD PRINTING

THE LIBRARY OF CONGRESS HAS CATALOGED THE HARDCOVER EDITION AS FOLLOWS:
Pollan, Michael.
A place of my own: the education of an amateur building / by Michael Pollan.
p. cm.
Includes index.
ISBN 0-679-41532-7 (hc.)
ISBN 978-0-14-311474-1 (pbk.)
1. Huts—Design and construction—Popular works.   2. Space and time—Popular works.   I. Title.
TH4890.P65   1997   690'.837—dc20   96-35101

Designed by J. K. Lambert
Title page photo copyright © 1997 by John Peden

For Isaac

"With this more substantial shelter about me, I had made some progress toward settling in the world."

—Henry David Thoreau, *Walden*

Preface

A *Place of My Own* is the biography of a building. In a sense it is the biography of every building, but happens to dwell on one in particular: the not-so-primitive hut I built in the woods behind my house in New England, as a place to read and write and daydream. This is not a famous or important building, but to me it has meant the world: I built it with my own two unhandy hands, and it is in here I wrote the book you now hold, as well as a second (*The Botany of Desire*) and a third of a third (*The Omnivore's Dilemma*).

But the book could have been written about almost any building because at its heart is a narrative of the universal process of design and construction—which is to say, the age-old story of how dreams get turned into drawings that then get turned into wood and stone and glass, finally to take their place in the palpable world. I have always found that process wonderful and slightly mysterious, and the people involved—architects and builders—particularly impressive characters. Architects do their work on the frontier between the ideal and the practical, translating wisps of ideas into buildable facts, and carpenters are among those lucky souls whose handiwork actually adds to the available stock of reality. To a writer, whose creations can really only be said to exist among the human speakers of his or her language, this is cause for envy. For us, terms like "architecture" and "carpentry" are little more than pretentious metaphors we use to dress up our far more ephemeral makings.

I had a dense tangle of reasons for wanting to build something, but one of them was to join the world of the makers—*homo faber*—and leave, if only temporarily, the dodgier world of words. I was looking for an antidote to the increasingly abstract and abstracted nature of my altogether typical working life, most of which was conducted in front of screens at an ever-greater remove from the natural world. It's possible I was also in the midst of a low-grade midlife crisis, and may have been looking for an escape hatch from a house that had mysteriously begun to shrink with the arrival of a new baby.

All this is true enough. But I also wanted very simply to learn how the work gets done: how exactly a designer goes about designing a successful space and a builder building it. At first I thought I could learn this by following the design and construction of a house or perhaps a skyscraper, and I started out on such a path. But I found I couldn't get as close to the subject and the work as I wanted to, and eventually realized I could learn a lot more by radically shrinking the dimensions of the project, stripping it down to its essentials and to a scale where I could work on it with my own hands right in my own backyard, as it were. In other words, I decided to conceive and build a microcosm: a place of my own that would also be a tool for exploring architecture.

It wasn't until I started down this path that I learned that the history of architecture contains a rich tradition of such microcosms—stories about elemental buildings conceived as a way to return architecture to its first principles. Beginning with the Primitive Hut described by the Roman architect and writer Vitruvius, accounts of the First Shelter have served as myths of the origins of architecture, as well as clever ways to argue for your particular view of how buildings should look and be built. Vitruvius' primitive hut looks a lot like a Greek temple built out of tree trunks and branches, thereby implying that the classical forms he admires were given to us by the forest itself, and so have the sanction of nature. Following his example, Alberti, Laugier, Frank

Lloyd Wright and Le Corbusier each constructed (at least in words) their own rhetorical hut as a way to argue for the naturalness or inevitability of their respective visions of architecture—neoclassical, Gothic, modern, whatever. In much the same way, many writers have built their own primitive huts—think of the ones in *Robinson Crusoe* or *Walden*—as a vantage from which to explore civilized man's relationship to nature and launch their critiques of modern society.

In retrospect I can see that my little cabin by the pond in Connecticut, and this account of it, is very much in the tradition of the Polemical Hut. In the course of its narrative, *A Place of My Own* puts forth an argument about architecture as well as modern life and work, all of which, I suggest, have lost the vital thread of their connection to nature, much to the detriment of our lives and buildings.

I mention all this because some readers (and even some reviewers) have approached *A Place of My Own* as a kind of how-to book that would tell them how to build their own cabin in the woods. I worry about those readers—and even more about their buildings. For while it's true that the book is organized, step-by-step, around the first-this-then-that syntax of designing and building a house, with chapters on Drawing, Foundations, Framing, Windows and Finishing, *A Place of My Own* was never intended as a recipe or construction manual. The book doesn't dwell quite long enough in the land of fig-1, fig-2 to insure that your own building will actually stand up or come out square. (Mine stands but as you will discover is, sadly, out of square.) *A Place of My Own* is not so much a how-to-do-it than a how-to-think-about-it kind of book.

≡

I have a theory that a writer's second book, which is what this one is for me, is the most difficult to write and the most revealing to read. To borrow a metaphor from geometry, a first book is like a point in the infinite space of literary possibility: it can be about anything and leads nowhere in particular. My first book, *Second Nature,* was ostensibly about my education as a gardener, and used the garden as a place to explore the complexities of our relationship to the natural world (including the peculiar fact that we have such a relationship; what other creature does?). But a writer's second book, by forming a second point in the space of literary possibility, creates a line: a path or trajectory that very often sets the course of the writer's career.

It is not until you embark on your second book that you begin to find out who you are as a writer. This happens in the course of discovering which of the questions that occupied you in the writing of your first book are dropped, and which turn out to be ones that you can't let go of. *A Place of My Own* is the book where that happened for me, and looking back I can see that in many ways it set me on my path.

When I embarked on *A Place of My Own* I thought I was leaving behind all the questions about nature and culture that had obsessed me in *Second Nature*. Now, I figured I was writing about a whole new set of questions having to do with architecture and building and work. After that, I presumably would turn my attention to another subject (politics? business? the Internet?), and then another.

But as I delved into the unfamiliar world of architecture, reading all I could about theories of design and the work of construction, visiting buildings, and learning how to read a plan and swing a hammer, something quite unexpected happened: I found myself drifting back to the same questions about nature and culture that had obsessed me during the writing of *Second Nature*. How do we humans fit into the natural world, and in what ways is that different from other creatures? Are our buildings the pure products of culture, like poems, or are they more like adaptations, akin to a pattern of camouflage in an animal? In what ways are our buildings like nests or burrows, the outcome of a kind of evolutionary process fitting our bodies and desires to the facts of our environment, and in what way are they free to be anything we like? In other words, does nature tell us how to build? Is the prestige of right angles or the Golden Section in Western architecture arbitrary, or is it rooted in something important about the nature of reality? Of course there are all sorts of other questions that come up in the process of designing and building, but these were the ones around which I kept circling.

For a while I struggled against the gravitational pull I felt dragging me back to nature, probably because in the back of every second-book writer looms this anxious injunction: *You don't want repeat yourself!* (That's just one of the many anxieties that don't disturb the sleep of the first-book writer.) This was the difficult part, and it sent me down many desolate narrative trails and up many thematically fruitless trees. But after several false starts, I came to the realization that these kinds of questions about nature were *my* question—the abiding ones that fired my curiosity and fed my imagination and about which I dared to hope I might have something useful to say. So maybe I wasn't repeating myself; maybe instead I was finding myself, or at least, finding the big questions that, for better or worse, would shape my work as a writer.

I suspect that every writer has some such set of ultimate questions, and if you read their work long enough you will find the path of their narrative or argument inevitably winding its way back to the Mother Issue, which might be power or money or sex, status or relationships or justice. Now I knew where my writing tended to gravitate and liked to linger: the messy places where the threads of nature and culture tangle in interesting ways. The reason I'd been drawn to writing about architecture in the first place was because architecture was, like gardens and agriculture and food, one of those interestingly messy places, where nature changes us even as we change nature. I was home.

≡

So *A Place of My Own* looks at the art of architecture and the work of building through the lens of nature. This was a decidedly idiosyncratic lens to deploy during the 1990s, when the book was written. For that was the decade when the architectural profession fell head over heels for literary theory, of all things, and was in the throes of a rebellion against the idea there was anything "natural" or necessary about a building, beyond the basic, boring necessity of keeping the rain off your client's head. (Not that it always succeeded at that.) Architect/theorists like Robert Venturi and Peter Eisenman held the microphone, and they were arguing in all sincerity that a building was in fact no different than a poem, that the conventions of architecture—things like gabled roofs and right angles—were just as arbitrary and culture-bound as the sounds of words in a language. Like words or letters, the meaning of these things derived not from facts of nature or the human body's experience of space but from the system of signs or the "language" of which they were a part.

In retrospect, the power of these ideas probably owed something to the fact that the Internet was just then making its presence felt in our lives, and the shiny possibilities of cyberspace seemed far more glamorous than old-fashioned physical spaces created out of bricks and mortar. At the time, transcending the limitations of nature, whatever you took them to be, seemed like an increasingly plausible and interesting project. For me, the irony of the situation was, well, inescapable. For just when I had turned to architecture and building in search of something more deeply rooted in reality than words, architects were giving all that up in order to be more like writers and software designers and sign-makers of every kind.

One of the things *A Place of My Own* attempts to do is to frame an argument against that conception of architecture, waging a defense of nature in the face of the glamour of all things digital and digitizable. In the years since the book was first published, architecture seems to have gotten over its most extreme literary conceits, and rediscovered the importance of such things as the body's experience of space. And yet in many ways, as our lives have grown ever more abstract and mediated, the book's defense of nature seems even more timely today than it did when it was written a decade ago.

≡

A Place of My Own ends with the completion of the building and the triumph of move-in day, but before I had taken up residence and gotten down to work. Many readers have written to ask what happened after that: did the writing house work out as I'd hoped? Do I still work in it? (They also write to ask where they might see photographs of the finished building. Go to my Web site, michaelpollan.com, and click on the image of the building on the home page.)

I had ten good years in my building before a move to California forced me, reluctantly, to abandon it. As I mentioned, I wrote two books and a portion of a third sitting at the broad ash desk looking out over the pond and garden. This proved to be a wonderful place to write and think and daydream, and in some ways the writing house exceeded my expectations. Except for the floor, the building is not insulated, so I assumed it would be only a seasonal place to work, but in fact I went to work in the writing house on all but the very bitterest or snowiest days. The two thick walls of books provided a measure of insulation, I suppose; the building was tight, I'm proud to say, and my little kerosene heater did a fine job of keeping the place nice and toasty. Snow was more likely to keep me away than cold, since there was a hundred-yard path between the house and the building that needed to be shoveled after a blizzard.

I loved that path, though, and the transition it afforded me as I strolled out to work every morning. My "commute" took only a few minutes, passing through the garden and under the arbor before winding around the pond and the building's companion boulder and then depositing me at the door. But in those few minutes, sipping from a mug of coffee and checking on my plants as I winded my way, I gradually shed the cares of the household and slipped back into the current of whatever it was I was writing. I would push open the door and crank up the heater, before stepping down into what I came to think of as my cockpit. Because once I took my seat at the desk, there was no reason whatsoever to move. Like a suit of clothes, Charlie had designed the space to the measure of my body, so everything I could possibly need—books, files, supplies, heater controls, machinery—I could reach without ever having to get up from my chair. Taking my seat in the lower section of the writing house came to feel like putting on a favorite old sweater or pair of socks. It fit me to a T.

Winter or summer, the building took on a completely different identity. Throwing open all the windows on an August afternoon—a ritual operation that involves hooking the two large in-swinging sashes to beams in the ceiling—instantly transformed the room into a screened-in porch. On a summer morning the room was delightful to work in, utterly transparent to the breeze and the sounds of birds and squirrels. But because the ceiling had no insulation, by three or so in the afternoon it sometimes got too warm to work. Oh well. The building was telling me to knock off, go for a swim, and so I did.

"First we shape our buildings," Winston Churchill famously said, "and thereafter our buildings shape us." I've often wondered how this building shaped me and my work in the years I did all my writing in it. Certainly the books and essays I wrote here were deeply rooted in the view from my desk, firmly planted in my garden. And since I've left the writing house my work has ventured farther afield from the garden I used to overlook and out into the wider world. Today the view from the room where I write includes the skyline of a city, so perhaps it isn't surprising that the writing might also have enlarged its purview, and grown a bit more political.

When the time came to move away, I gave some serious thought to putting the writing house on a flatbed truck and bringing it with me to California. But as you will soon learn, the building was as carefully fitted to its site as it was to me, and it's hard to imagine it displaced to an urban backyard in Berkeley. So in 2003 when we pulled up stakes in New England it stayed behind.

But though I may have abandoned the writing house, I couldn't bear to sell it or the house. So when we moved west we leased the place to a young couple who, like we do, work at home. Bill now works in the writing house, which he's put to a very different purpose. Bill manages real estate for living, and has filled the little building with steel file cabinets and more office equipment—photocopiers, faxes, printers, shredders—than I would have thought it could ever hold. There's a high-speed Internet connection now, and the place, which I try to check in on every summer, has a completely different feel to it. With the daybed piled high with file folders, the space for daydreaming has shrunk down to a cramped couple of square feet or so. What it feels like now is a crowded real-estate office plopped down in the woods.

I miss it sorely and look forward to the day when I'll be able to reclaim it and work in the writing house again. Still, I do spend a fair amount of imaginary time there, which is not nothing. Very often when I'm having trouble sleeping, or fretting over a sentence that refuses to unknot, or corralling a paragraph to go where I want it to, I'll put myself at the big ash desk, with the windows hitched up in August mode, and feel the soft breeze of a summer morning passing through the space. *A place of my own:* as it began it is once again, which is to say a cherished daydream. It is one I can usually count on to clear out my head, so I guess you could say I still get some good work done there, in the hut by the pond three thousand miles away.

Acknowledgments

I had a great deal of help in the making of *A Place of My Own*—both the building and the book. I can't imagine a better guide to the world of architecture than Charles Myer, or to the world of carpentry than Joe Benney—these friends, my Virgils, were the best of teachers and companions. Besides giving me an education in the intricacies of their respective crafts, Charlie and Joe both read the manuscript and made valuable suggestions.

Mark Edmundson read several drafts of the book and never failed to improve it by his comments; I felt him by my side at every step. I was also fortunate to have the wise and generous editorial help of Allan Gurganus and Mark Danner. Ileene Smith read the final draft with scrupulous care; only another writer who has had the benefit of her judgment and her ear can know the value of her contribution.

In Ann Godoff I have everything a writer could ask for in an editor: wisdom, encouragement, patience, and friendship. Amanda Urban, my agent, was not only unflagging in her enthusiasm, as always, but also inspired in her editorial suggestions. My thanks, too, to Elsa Burt, Enrica Gadler, Jim Evangelisti, Don Knerr, Susan Dunbar, Don Statham, Jessica Green, Gerald Marzorati, Dominique Browning, Malka Margolies, Christopher Stamey, and Liz Denton.

But, finally, it is Judith to whom I owe this book. There is not a page in it that doesn't bear the mark of her thoughtfulness, encouragement, and sacrifice. Though Judith made it a point never to hit a single nail, neither the book nor the building would stand if not for her generosity. In more ways than I can say, *A Place of My Own* is her gift.

Contents

Preface ix

Acknowledgments xix

Chapter 1: A Room of One's Own 3

Chapter 2: The Site 30

Chapter 3: On Paper 53

Chapter 4: Footings 99

Chapter 5: Framing 132

Chapter 6: The Roof 176

Chapter 7: Windows 223

Chapter 8: Finish Work 267

Sources 303

Index 311

A Place of My Own

CHAPTER 1

A Room
of One's Own

A room of one's own: Is there anybody who hasn't
at one time or another wished for such a place,
hasn't turned those soft words over until they'd assumed a habitable shape? What they propose, to
anyone who admits them into the space of a daydream, is a place of solitude a few steps off the
beaten track of everyday life. Beyond that, though,
the form the dream takes seems to vary with the
dreamer. Generally the imagined room has a fixed
terrestrial address, whether located deep within
the family house or out in the woods under its own
roof. For some people, though, the same dream
can just as easily assume a vehicular form. I'm
thinking of the one-person cockpit or cabin, a mobile room in which to journey some distance from

the shore of one's usual cares. Fixed or mobile, a dream of escape is what this probably sounds like. But it's more like a wish for a slightly different angle on things—for the view from the tower, or tree line, or the bobbing point a couple hundred yards off the coast. It might be a view of the same old life, but from out here it will look different, the outlines of the self a little more distinct.

In my own case, there came a moment—a few years shy of my fortieth birthday, and on the verge of making several large changes in my life—when the notion of a room of my own, and specifically, of a little wood-frame hut in the woods behind my house, began to occupy my imaginings with a mounting insistence. This in itself didn't surprise me particularly. I was in the process of pulling my life up by the roots, all at once becoming a father, leaving the city where I'd lived since college, and setting out on an uncertain new career. Indeed, it would have been strange if I *hadn't* entertained fantasies of escape or, as I preferred to think of it, *simplification*— of reducing so many daunting new complexities to something as stripped-down and uncomplicated as a hut in the woods. What was surprising, though, and what had no obvious cause or explanation in my life as it had been lived up to then, was a corollary to the dream: I wanted not only a room of my own, but a room of my own making. I wanted to build this place myself.

To know me even slightly is to know how ill-equipped I was to undertake such an enterprise, and how completely out of character it would be. Like my father—who only very briefly owned a toolbox, and who regarded the ethic of the do-it-yourselfer as about as alien as Zen—I am a radically unhandy man for whom the hanging of a picture or the changing of a washer is a fairly big deal. To Judith, my wife, I am "the Jewish fix-it man"—this being a contradiction in terms, a creature no more plausible than a unicorn. Apart from eating, gardening, short-haul driving, and sex, I generally preferred to delegate my commerce with the physical world to specialists; things seemed to work out better that way. Unnecessary physical tests hold no romance for me, and I am not ordinarily given to Thoreauvian fantasies of self-sufficiency or worries about the fate of manhood in the modern world. I'm a writer and editor by trade, more at home in the country of words than things.

At home, perhaps, yet not entirely content, and in this dim restlessness may lie a clue to the unexpected emergence of my do-it-yourself self. For if the wish for a room of my own answered to a need I felt for a literal and psychic space, the wish to build it with my own hands, though slower to surface, may have reflected some doubts I was having about the sort of work I do. Work is how we situate ourselves in the world, and like the work of many people nowadays, mine put me in a relationship to the world that often seemed abstract, glancing, secondhand. Or thirdhand, in my case, for I spent much of my day working on other peoples' words, *re*writing, *re*vising, *re*wording. Oh, it was real work (I guess), but it didn't always feel that way, possibly because there were whole parts of me it failed to address. (Like my body, with the exception of the carpal tunnel in my wrist.) Nor did what I do seem to add much, if anything, to the stock of reality, and though this might be a dated or romantic notion in an age of information, it seemed to me this was something real work should do. Whenever I heard myself described as an "information-services worker" or a "symbolic analyst," I wanted to reach for a hammer, or a hoe, and with it make something less virtual than a sentence.

But the do-it-myself part came later; first came the wish for the space—specifically, for a simple, one-room outbuilding where I could write and read outside the house, at least during the summer months. Even after a substantial renovation, our house is tiny, and as Judith's due date approached, it seemed to grow tinier still. As our rooms filled up with the bassinet and booster seat, the crib and high chair and changing table, the walker and stroller and bouncer and monitor, a house that had always seemed a distinct reflection of two individuals living a particular life in a particular place began to feel more like some sort of franchise, a generic nonplace furnished in white polyethylene and licensed fictional beings. Whatever the virtues of such an environment for raising a child, it was not one where I could easily imagine reading a book without pictures in it through to the end, much less getting one written.

Probably this sounds like nothing more than the panic of a new father, and I don't discount that, but there were other factors at work here too. At roughly the same time, I was preparing to give up my office in the city, where I had a job at a magazine, to begin working out of my house, writing full-time. My office had never been much to look at—it was a standard corporate cube in a "sick building" with toxic air. Even so, it was a space where I enjoyed a certain sovereignty, where I could shut my door and maintain my desk in a state easily mistaken for chaos, and I was giving it up at the very moment that my house was shrinking. As for Judith, she already had a room of her own—the studio where she went each day to paint in perfect solitude. Now even this cluttered and fumy barn became a place I gazed at longingly.

I too needed a place to work. That at least is the answer I had prepared for anybody who asked what exactly I was doing out there in the woods with my hammer and circular saw for what turned out to be two and a half years of Sundays. I was building an office for myself, an enterprise so respectable that the federal government gives you tax deductions for it.

But the official home-office answer, while technically accurate and morally unimpeachable, doesn't tell the whole story of why I wanted a room of my own in the woods, a dream that, in its emotional totality, fits awkwardly onto the lines of a 1040 form, not to mention those of casual conversation. I was glad to have a sensible-sounding explanation I could trot out when necessary, but what I felt the need for was not nearly so rational, and much more difficult to name.

It was right around this time that I stumbled upon a French writer named Gaston Bachelard, a brilliant and sympathetic student of the irrational, who helped me to locate some of the deeper springs of my wish. "If I were asked to name the chief benefits of the house," Bachelard wrote in a beautiful, quirky 1958 book called *The Poetics of Space*, "I should say: the house shelters daydreaming, the house protects the dreamer, the house allows one to dream in peace." An obvious idea perhaps, but in it I recognized at once what it was I'd lost and dreamt of recovering.

Daydreaming does not enjoy tremendous prestige in our culture, which tends to regard it as unproductive thought. Writers perhaps appreciate its importance better than most, since a fair amount of what they call work consists of little more than daydreaming edited. Yet anyone who reads for pleasure should prize it too, for what is reading a good book but a daydream at second hand? Unlike any other form of thought, daydreaming is its own reward. For regardless of the result (if any), the very process of daydreaming is pleasurable. And, I would guess, is probably a psychological necessity. For isn't it in our daydreams that we acquire some sense of what we are about? Where we try on futures and practice our voices before committing ourselves to words or deeds? Daydreaming is where we go to cultivate the self, or, more likely, selves, out of the view and earshot of other people. Without its daydreams, the self is apt to shrink down to the size and shape of the estimation of others.

To daydream obviously depends on a certain degree of solitude, but I didn't always appreciate that it might require its own literal and dedicated place. For isn't walking or driving to work or waiting on line for the ATM space enough in which to daydream? Not deeply or freely, according to Bachelard; true reverie needs a physical shelter, though the architectural requirements he sets forth for it are slight. In Bachelard's view the room of one's own need be nothing more than an attic or basement, a comfortable winged chair off in the corner, or even the circle of contemplative space created by a fire in a hearth. In *A Room of One's Own*, Virginia Woolf sets more stringent specifications for the space, probably because she is concerned with one particular subset of daydreamer—

the female writer—whose requirements are somewhat greater on account of the demands often made on her by others. "A lock on the door," Woolf writes, "means the power to think for oneself."

Both Woolf and Bachelard are obviously writing as moderns, for the notion of a room of one's own—a place of solitude for the individual—is historically speaking a fairly recent invention. But then again, so is the self, or at least the self as we've come to think of it, an individual with a rich interior life. Dipping recently into a multivolume history of private life edited by Philippe Ariès, I was fascinated to learn how the room of one's own (specifically, the private study located off the master bedroom) and the modern sense of the individual emerged at more or less the same moment during the Renaissance. Apparently this is no accident: The new space and the new self actually helped give shape to one another. It appears there is a kind of reciprocity between interiors and interiority.

The room of one's own that Woolf and Bachelard and the French historians all talked about as necessary to the interior life was located firmly within the confines of a larger house, whether it was an attic nook, a locked room, or a study off the master bedroom. I shared that dream, as far as it went. But none of these images quite squared with my own, which featured not only four walls but also a roof and several windows filled with views of the woods and fields. Not just a room, it was a *building* of my own I wanted, an outpost of solitude pitched somewhere in the landscape rather than in the house. And so I began to wonder (not one to leave any such thing unexamined) where in the world could *that* part of the dream have come from? Who, in other words, put a roof on it?

≡

The deepest roots of such a dream are invariably obscure, a tangle of memories and circumstances, things read in books and pictures glimpsed in magazines. But the simplest answer to that question is an architect by the name of Charles R. Myer, an old friend from my college days whose off-hand suggestion set this whole project in motion. Though that was the very last thing I would have expected at the time, since I had dismissed the suggestion out of hand, deeming it tactless and quite possibly insane.

It was Charlie Myer who'd helped us renovate our tiny bungalow in the northwest corner of Connecticut, where most of this story takes place. It is, or at least it was, a resolutely nondescript clapboard house built in the 1930s from a Sears, Roebuck mail-order kit by a farmer named Matyas. The house is tucked into a roadside corner of an obstreperous wedge of land that climbs and leaps up the rocky hillside behind it like an unwieldy green kite. Not surprisingly, this land eventually defeated the farmer, but in the years since we'd moved in and begun to reclaim the remaining few acres of his falling-down dairy farm from the forest's encroachment, we'd grown unreasonably attached to the place. I say "unreasonably" because any truly sensible person would have moved rather than attempt to rescue a house as ordinary and unsound as this one.

I mention all this because the beginning of this story—the inception of my building—takes place in the midst of this renovation, at a second-story bedroom window that looks back toward the hillside. It was in April, I believe, and the renovation of the house was at long last approaching completion, after a year so emotionally trying and financially devastating that I still don't like to talk about it. We were not out of the woods quite yet—the new second floor had been framed, roofed, and clad in plywood, but the window in question was still nothing more than a rough opening to the air outlined in two-by-six studs.

On good days that year, Judith and I regarded Charlie with gratitude and even a measure of awe: it was already evident he had succeeded in transforming our humdrum little bungalow into a house of real character and, for us then, what seemed a perfect fit. On certain other days, however, when the complexity of Charlie's design had brought our contractor to the cliff of despair and move-in day had retreated yet another month, I eyed Charlie with suspicion, if not outright fear, seriously wondering whether this man wasn't really Ahab disguised as an architect, piloting us all toward certain ruin in quest of some dubious ideal only he completely understood.

But on this particular April morning I was taking the more benign view, at least to start. After going completely roofless for the better part of March, our bedroom was at last starting to resemble a room. Charlie was down from Cambridge on one of his monthly site inspections; when I arrived, his Trooper was already beached in the crisscrossed field of mud that had formerly been our front lawn. His car looked lived in, its backseat buried beneath a heap of rolled-up blueprints, action figures (Charlie has two boys), Styrofoam coffee cups, and wadded cigarette packs. After climbing the contractor's rickety extension ladder and stepping out onto the new plywood subfloor, I saw Charlie's bearish frame in the new window opening; clomping from one boot to the other to keep warm, he was peering out at the early spring landscape, still only incipiently green, with a cigarette cupped in his hand. This was the first time either of us had had the chance to glimpse what amounted to an entirely fresh perspective on the property—the startlingly new landscape a well-placed window can create. One of the aims of Charlie's design had been to redirect the house's gaze away from the road in front and back toward the hillside and our gardens, and it was clear from here that he had succeeded.

Charlie greeted me with his customary "Hey," a quick throaty bark he somehow manages to work some warmth into. He immediately dropped his cigarette, grinding it into the plywood with his boot. I've told him maybe a half-dozen times his smoking doesn't bother me, and anyway the "room" we were standing in was wide open to the weather, but Charlie likes to think of himself as someone who's quit, so he allows himself to smoke only in the car or outdoors, and then only when alone. This was an accommodation that seemed very much in character, especially in the way it carefully layered an intricate regime of self-discipline over the absence of that very quality. In Charlie the supreme self-control and orderliness I associate with architects seems to be at constant loggerheads with deeper forces and appetites that he is too much a creature of the senses to master completely.

It is a contest that is perhaps most openly waged in his attire, which despite his best efforts invariably puts you in mind of a hastily made bed. This morning, for example, Charlie had on under his suede jacket a very sharp new J. Crew shirt, but already it was climbing up out of his chinos, which were themselves riding alarmingly low. The man's rumpledness is so deep-seated it would probably defeat Armani, assuming Charlie could afford such tailoring; he's just too baggy and lumbering a guy. He's also too much of a Yankee: Charlie's the kind of New Englander (he grew up in Cambridge, in a family of Quakers that came to Massachusetts in 1650) for whom the absolute worst thing you can say about someone, or something, is that it's pretentious.

Not that this makes him the least bit careless about his presentation; to the contrary, Charlie has the architect's clichéd self-consciousness about image and sensitivity to detail; it's just that he's loathe to come across that way. In fact he considers it a high compliment whenever a client tells him he doesn't seem like an architect, since what people usually mean by this is that he listens well, is practical-minded, and prizes comfort as much as beauty. (*Comf'table*, pronounced in a cushy three-syllable version, is a favorite word; so is *neat*, deployed strictly as a superlative.) And, anyway, with two hundred hirsute pounds distributed somewhat unevenly over a six-foot frame, and a face of unusual sympathy and expressiveness—it's animated by a footloose pair of shrubby eyebrows that almost touch in the middle—Charlie doesn't look the part. But though the tail of his shirt may be on the loose, marching across his breast pocket you will invariably find a serried rank of pens and markers, their arrangement as fixed as the stars. I once asked him how his little system worked. "System?" he stammered. "You've got the wrong architect!" Yet after the gentlest prod he spelled it out in detail: "So, okay, the felt-tip here in first position? That's a Stylist, for taking notes during meetings. Next up's the black Expresso Bold, for rough schematic drawings, your basic big picture stuff, followed by the colored marker—usually red, but sometimes green—which I use to indicate clients' changes on working drawings. And last but not least, the classic black Uniball fine-point, which is reserved exclusively for drafting." Inside a very human exterior lurks the soul of an architect struggling to get out.

It eventually became clear that, on this particular morning, the architect was in fact out and about. Charlie seemed pleased with the new room and its windows, but I could tell that something in this picture was bugging him. When I asked him what it was, he tried to demur, but his eyebrows had started to dance. One of the errors in Charlie's self-conception is that he's extremely good at hiding his feelings.

I pressed, and he pointed out the window at the view.

Looking out the bedroom window, you could follow the informal axis along which our garden had developed, as we gradually extended a slender finger of civilization from the back door out into what Judith had taken to calling the Wilderness: the irrepressible second-growth forest and scrub that was steadily marching down the hillside, threatening to engulf what was left of the farm and the little house. At ground level, from the old first-floor windows, this narrow corridor of grass with its adjoining beds of flowers, its rose arbor and fieldstone walls, had seemed a genuine accomplishment. But from here our hard-won path out into the land seemed more tenuous and paltry than I'd remembered it, and I guessed this was what was troubling Charlie about the view. The axis was all but lost in the big, turbulent landscape framed by the new window, expiring abruptly just past the arbor, which now seemed a few short steps from the back door. A nice pie of meadow was now visible in the distance, part way up the hillside, but the path held out no hope of ever reaching it. Suddenly it looked pointless. The elevated view Charlie had created had diminished the scope of the garden, and with it the reassuring marks of our presence in this landscape. We were back where we'd started more than a decade ago, the little house cowering behind its moat of lawn, struggling to fend off the advancing forest.

What the garden's axis needed now, the architect had concluded, was a destination—some sort of distinct object in the distance that would draw your eye out into the land and up the hill, somehow tie the cultivated foreground into the larger landscape above. I could sort of see his point, but it seemed to me this particular problem belonged down near the very bottom of a to-do list that had grown dauntingly tall. Judith and I were still camped out at my parents'.

"So you mean like a bench or something?"

"That would help. Absolutely. But I've got a neater idea." He looked at me and grinned slightly, trying to gauge my appetite for neat new ideas, the last set not having yet been completely digested or paid for. "What I think we need to do is build something out there," he began, extending an index finger through the rough opening and wagging it in the general direction of the meadow. "I haven't figured out exactly what yet, but I think—in fact I *know*—that a little structure somewhere out there could really, really work. You need to think about it."

Just then I doubt there was anything I wanted to think about less. The prospect of embarking on any new construction project was so far out of the question as to be laughable. Our contractor was running four months behind schedule, he'd just admitted that he had no idea where to find the "neat" postage-stamp-size windows Charlie had spec'd for the gable ends, or how in the world he was ever going to bend a four-by-four piece of lumber to form the porch's "neat" curving lintels. Our savings had been cleaned out, and we were about to return to the bank for a second mortgage. The very last thing we needed now was another neat idea from Charlie.

I decided the best thing to do was just to let the suggestion lie, even after Charlie, warming to his plan, offered to design the new building free of charge. I didn't know whether to regard this as an act of generosity from a friend or a particularly flagrant case of the monomania to which members of his profession seem to be prone. The odd thing about it was, I had never thought of Charlie that way. Compared to the Ayn Rand stereotype of the architect as a power-mad empire builder, a chilly figure at home only in the realm of his own ideal forms, Charlie had always seemed to me a fairly contented citizen of the real world, somebody with a deep appreciation for life as it is really lived, in all its unplatonic messiness. Yet here he was, actually suggesting that what the view from the window of his new building needed most of all was another Charlie Myer building.

I thanked him for the generous offer and promptly changed the subject to something compelling, like plumbing fixtures.

≡

But I guess the notion had been planted, because many months later, when my thoughts turned to a room of my own, I found it was from the bedroom window that I invariably imagined it. Eventually I constructed a fairly detailed little daydream about the place, in which I followed myself walking down the garden path on a dewy summer morning with a cup of coffee in my hand, stepping under the rose arbor, ambling up the hill into the woods, and eventually coming upon my hut, which was planted somewhere far enough from the road that the world outside its door faded to rumor. What did the hut look like? The particulars were indistinct, except that the building seemed more woodsy than the house. It was shingled rather than clapboarded, for example, and had a steeply sloped gable roof.

Rehearsing this scenario in bed late one night, during one of the frequent bouts of sleeplessness I credited to incipient fatherhood, it occurred to me that my image of the building was based at least partly on a tree house I'd had as a child, growing up on Long Island—the last time I'd had a room of my own off in the woods. Strictly speaking, this wasn't a tree house, since there were no trees involved in its construction, at least not living ones. It was more like a little cape on stilts, a gable-roofed room maybe ten feet by six, and raised five feet off the ground on four pressure-treated posts. My father had hired a contractor named Goeltz to build it for me. Together they'd knocked off the design from a picture of a fancy playhouse my father and I had admired in the Hammacher Schlemmer catalog.

The reason I didn't have a normal, dad-built tree house is that, as I've indicated, I didn't have anything even approaching that kind of dad. He was, and remains, one of the world's great indoorsmen, a delegator of all conceivable outdoor tasks—lawn mowing, car washing, gutter cleaning, and tree-house building. By the time I was ten, which was when I'd kicked off my campaign for a tree house in the woods behind our ranch, he didn't even own the tools needed to build one, having "accidentally" nailed his tool chest behind the walls of a cedar closet he'd tried to build for my mother in the basement. Whether consciously or not, my father had clearly wanted to make sure the cedar closet would be his last do-it-yourself project, and it was.

Not that I'm complaining, because it was due solely to his confirmed unhandiness that I ended up with the fanciest tree house in the development, one that boasted a pair of shuttered windows, a pine-plank floor, and a shingled roof. But the very best thing about my tree house (and the thing about it that, as a parent now myself, I find most astounding) was that no one but a kid could possibly gain admittance to it: the only way in was by climbing up a flimsy rope ladder and squeezing through a trapdoor in the floor that couldn't have been more than eighteen inches square. As much as the tree house itself, the tiny trapdoor was a gift of extraordinary generosity: my parents had underwritten my dream of a place from which even they would be excluded.

Arguably this was a foolish thing for them to do, because later on the tree house would serve as the setting for various illicit activities. Though even then, it all seemed something less than authentically depraved—a matter of symbolism mainly, not that that was unimportant. Paging through a *Playboy* or smoking pot up in the tree house, the point was in many ways less sexual or pharmacological than sacramental, odd as that might sound. For this was high childhood ritual, and more than anything else, it was the tree house itself that these ceremonies commemorated, this airborne room of my own, which I came to regard as a temple of my privacy and independence.

≡

Even more than adults do, children seem instinctively to grasp the deepest meanings of *houseness*—the full significance of territory and shelter, the metaphysics of inside and out, the symbolism of doors and windows and roofs. Shelter, for example, is a concept that nothing could underline as emphatically as a hail of well-thrown rocks. When I read *Beowulf* in college, all those vivid scenes of the mead hall under siege from Grendel made me think of those first thrilling nights my friends and I spent sleeping out in the new tree house, withstanding the predawn assaults of our enemies. Our local Grendel was an older boy named Jeff Grabel, who took it upon himself to terrorize us for reasons that were never articulated, but which we spent hours speculating about. The prevailing theory held that the dispute was territorial, since the tree house had been built in the middle of the half-acre wood that sep-

arated his family's house from mine. Though this property technically belonged to my family, Grabel had had the run of it before the
construction of the tree house, so it made sense he would have regarded our outpost as an alien incursion. For more than a year he
dedicated his every effort to erasing our presence from the woods
while we, with a matching tenacity, dedicated ours to preserving a
toehold.

"Every child begins the world again," Thoreau wrote in *Walden,*
and it's certainly true that the games of boys can be almost car-
toonishly atavistic, dredging up from who-knows-where the primordial struggles of the race. Between Grabel and me the cause
was nothing less than that of chaos against civilization, Grendel
against the mead hall, the Sioux against the settler. (The first time
I had occasion to meet Jeff Grabel off the field of battle, years later,
I was surprised to find he could form an English sentence; during
raids he had whooped exclusively.) The symbol of civilization we'd
set out to defend was my little stilt-house in the woods, four walls
and a gable roof, its archetypal form signifying home, settlement,
and in the context of that forest, defiance. The hearth around
which we gathered after dark was a flashlight, whose beam reflecting down off the ceiling held us in a warm circle of light. For mead
we had cans of Hawaiian Punch. And outside all around us chaos
raged.

Grabel and his allies chucked stones that would thud against the
wood walls of the tree house with enough force to rock it on its
posts. We would retaliate with water balloons, frequently delivered
by catapult. Usually we felt fairly safe up there in the trees, the
house's windows shuttered against the hail of stones, but Grabel
could keep it up all night, and sometimes we'd begin to feel
trapped. Climbing down out of the tree house before dawn for any
reason was out of the question. And this was occasionally a problem, as when one of us had to pee during the night. At first we relied on the equivalent of a bedpan, but this did not accord with the

warrior image we were cultivating, so eventually we devised a more satisfactory solution: a curved length of black plastic pipe slipped through a knothole in the wall. The beauty of this appliance was that it could double as a weapon: its range and trajectory were adjustable to some degree, and we could hear Grabel scramble for cover whenever the long black snout emerged from its slot.

The tree house was always at its best under siege, creaking in the wind, its posts bending slightly, the better to withstand the blows. Bachelard says that this is a property of houses in general, that they only come into their own in bad weather, when the poetry of shelter receives its fullest expression. A house under siege from the elements becomes "an instrument with which to confront the cosmos," he writes. "Come what may the house helps us to say: I will be an inhabitant of the world, in spite of the world."

≡

That was at night. During the day Grabel slept (or went to elementary school), and the significance of the tree house shifted. Instead of serving as a battleground, the building became a safer, more solitary, and dreamier place, my rural retreat from the cares of the big ranch house where, nominally, I lived with my three sisters, two parents, and numberless pets. Yet the tree house was in fact not the first such retreat I'd had. Even this room had its precursors, though these were strictly ad hoc and sited within the walls of my parent's house. I'm thinking of the huts a child builds with an appliance carton, or two chairs and a blanket, or of one particular closet I cleared of coats and outfitted (with dials and gauges drawn in Magic Marker) to resemble a Gemini capsule. (NASA's ingenious, high-tech envelopes of space have probably inflected my notion of the ideal room since the first time I watched Jules Bergman fold himself into one on television.) Lori, the oldest of my sisters, kept house for a time in another closet directly beneath the basement stairs, which gave the space a steeply sloped roof, lending it the feel of a cottage. Though these huts were firmly held in the embrace of our parent's house, they formed another interior deep inside it, a second, more comprehensible frontier of inside and out, private and public, self and world, that we children could control.

Bachelard's *The Poetics of Space* is the only book I've ever read that takes these sorts of places seriously, analyzing them—or at least our memories and dreams of them—as a way to understand our deepest, most subjective experience of place. He suggests that our sense of space is organized around two distinct poles, or tropisms: one attracting us to the vertical (compelling us to seek the power and rationality of the tower view) and the other to the enclosed center, what he sometimes calls the "hut dream." It is this second, centripetal attractor that inspires the child to build imaginary huts under tabletops and deep inside coat closets, and draws the adult toward the hearth or the kitchen table, places of maximum refuge that hold us in a small, concentrated circle of warmth. These, in Bachelard's terms, are huts too.

Of course Bachelard, a Frenchman, is describing a European's sense of space, and an American—especially an American with childhood memories of a tree house and a quasi-adult dream of building a hut in the woods—can't help but wonder if maybe we experience space somewhat differently in this country. For in addition to the centripetal impulse that Bachelard so tenderly describes—our wish to be "enclosed, protected, all warm in the bosom of the house"—isn't there also a centrifugal impulse at work in the American dream of houses, one that is always pushing us outward, flinging open windows and reaching out into the surrounding landscape?

One of the all-time great American houses—and one that no doubt stands behind any American's wish for a room of one's own—exhibits exactly this quality, at least in its author/architect/builder's description of it. At Walden, after procrastinating for most of the summer of 1845, Henry David Thoreau finally built a hearth in time for winter, but he always seems much less enamored of his house's sense of enclosure than of its unusual transparency. He delights every time a sparrow or a field mouse manages to infiltrate his cabin, which appears to have been no great feat. Thoreau waited until the freezing weather of November before he plastered the interior, so much did he enjoy the free passage of wind and sunlight through the knotholes and chinks in his walls.

With his cabin "so slightly clad," Thoreau wrote, "I did not need to go out doors to take the air, for the atmosphere within had lost none of its freshness. It was not so much within doors as behind a door where I sat, even in the rainiest weather." It's almost as though Thoreau's dream house keeps wanting to dissolve itself back into the landscape; he cannot make his walls thin enough, and has nothing but scorn for the whole hypercivilized distinction between inside and out. What he calls his "best room," in fact, was no room at all, but the "pine wood behind my house. Thither in summer days, when distinguished guests came, I took them, and a priceless domestic swept the floor and dusted the furniture and kept the things in order."

However whimsical, Thoreau was giving voice to a concept of American space that others of a slightly more practical bent would eventually pick up on. Indeed, it could be argued that Thoreau's crude hut by the pond, or at least his account of it, has had a profound impact on the course of American architecture. Certainly Thoreau was militating for a transparency to nature and an open plan—for "a house whose inside is as open and manifest as a bird's nest"—long before American architecture attempted to build these things.

The modernist glass house eventually fulfilled Thoreau's dream of transparency—and brought its inhumanness to light. For although the glass house was a brilliant conceit, the material embodiment of the American romance of nature, it proved to be an inhospitable shelter. It fell to Frank Lloyd Wright to realize Thoreau's dream of a centrifugal house without forsaking the satisfactions of shelter that Bachelard describes. Wright designed houses with strong, compelling centers ("It comforted me," he said in accounting for his love of massive central hearths, "to see the fire burning deep in the solid masonry of the house itself") that nevertheless unfolded outward, pushing into the surrounding landscape and dematerializing their walls—metaphorically scraping off Thoreau's regretted plaster in order to admit nature once again, though on our own terms now. Outdoor nature for Bachelard is something the archetypal house girds against, or offers refuge from. For Thoreau and Wright and generations of American house builders, the land is what the house wants to embrace.

≡

It must have been some such sense of American space that compelled me to situate my dream of a hut out in the woods, first as a child and then, some thirty years on, as a parent-to-be. Being the most literal people the world has ever known, it's hard to imagine any American possessed by such a dream contenting himself for very long with the sort of imaginary hut-within-the-house Bachelard describes. Or even, for that matter, with Virginia Woolf's room of one's own, since her room is not a built thing so much as an agreed-upon thing, a consensual space located within a house still under the control of others. We Americans have always taken our metaphors very seriously, ever since we first decided it would be a good idea to site and actually build the "city on a hill" that generations of less literal-minded people had been content to regard as a nice figure of speech. But giving form and an address to our most abstract mental constructs—to our wildest dreams—seems to be what we do here. "Build therefore your own world," Emerson urged, and we have tried.

This doesn't, however, quite explain how my own grown-up dream of a hut expanded to include the improbable idea of building it with my own hands. Any number of qualified general contractors could have rendered my dream perfectly literal with no help from me, and I'm sure it would have turned out a lot more square and true than it did. This was the part—the do-it-yourself part—that I could not have foreseen. Judith suspects that the prospect of a house vibrating with the howls of an infant—our son, Isaac, was born shortly before construction began—would have made any time-consuming outdoor project look attractive just then. Maybe, but you'd think I could have come up with an easier and more socially acceptable avenue of escape, like taking on paid work for which I had some acumen.

At least some of the blame for this unlikely turn of events should probably go to a captivating if slightly irresponsible book that Charlie lent me soon after our fateful exchange before the bedroom window. The book was called *Tiny Houses*, and had been written, or drawn (since it contains very few words), by an architect by the name of Lester Walker. Essentially a pattern book, and very much in the American grain, *Tiny Houses* presents photographs and architectural drawings of some forty one-person structures. The book includes plans for most of the tiny houses I knew about—Thoreau's cabin; Jefferson's honeymoon cottage (where he lived for several years while Monticello was being built); George Bernard Shaw's writing hut—and a great many others I didn't. There are ice-fishing shanties built on top of frozen lakes; a handful of funky prefab cottages; a forty-two-square-foot "rolling home" built in the back of a 1949 delivery van; several minuscule vacation cabins (including an "inside-out" summer house in which everything but the bed is arranged along the *exterior* walls of a tiny sleeping hut—perhaps the ultimate centrifugal house); a self-sufficient mobile home modeled on a space capsule (!); a two-hole outhouse that a painter had converted into a meditation hut, and, the tiniest house of all, a wooden bus shelter that measures two feet four inches square and can hold two children "but only if they are standing."

As Charlie may very well have hoped, I found myself spending a fair number of my insomniac hours in the company of *Tiny Houses*, marveling at the ingenuity of their designs, the enterprise of their builders, and more than anything else, the distinct and exceedingly quirky character of these structures. The best of them were houses cast in the first-person singular, each the precise material expression, in wood or canvas or aluminum or plastic or simple tar paper, of a single individual. By studying the plans and snapshots of these houses you felt you understood something essential about their builders, as though the building were a second face, another window on the self. After paying a visit to his friend Daniel Ricketson's vine-tangled Gothic Revival shanty in Brooklawn, Massachusetts, Thoreau wrote in his journal that in the building's architecture "I found all his peculiarities faithfully expressed, his humanity, his fear of death, love of retirement, simplicity, etc."

I doubt that a big house could ever offer quite so intense a distillation of a single character or voice, so tight and uncompromising a fit of space to self. George Bernard Shaw's writing hut, for example, an eight-by-eight pine shack at the bottom of his garden, was constructed on a steel turntable that allowed him to single-handedly rotate the building during the course of the day, in order to follow the arc of the sun. What could better suit a playwright than a house that looked at the world not from any one angle, but from every possible angle in turn?

Books like this have a way of gently interrogating the reader's imagination, provoking the kinds of questions that can only be answered by way of a daydream. One cannot skim *Tiny Houses* without wondering, What would *my* first-person house look like? Would it be fixed or mobile, and what should it be made of? Where's the best place to site it, and what would I want its windows to look out on? And yet there is one fairly obvious question the book plainly doesn't want you to ask, which is, Who could I hire to build it for me?

"One of the great thrills in life is to inhabit a building that one has built oneself," Walker writes in his introduction, neatly closing off that particular avenue of speculation. "My goal was to inspire people of all ages and degrees of carpentry skill . . . to take hammer in hand and build themselves a little dream." There was something intrinsically do-it-yourself about the best of these buildings. You could see how their character was part and parcel of the work that went into making them, work that bore all the marks of the amateur. And one of those marks, as that word's root reminds us, is love.

A house in the first person did not seem like something a third party could build. To hire the local Goeltz, to knock the thing off from a picture in a catalog, was to miss the point, or at least, the possibility. For besides getting his son off his back for a while, what had my father really gotten out of his hut-building project? What had he learned from it? Not nearly as much as he might have, or as I stood to were I to build my house myself. I began to see how there might be a connection between the kind of mental life I hoped such a place might house and the kind of work I'd have to learn in order to build it, a connection hinted at in words such as *independence, individual, pragmatic, self-made.* To build a house in the first person, a place as much one's own as a second skin, would require an exploration of self and place—and work itself—that simply could not be delegated to somebody else. The meaning of such a place was in its making.

And anyway, this Lester Walker made building sound so easy, so roll-up-your-sleeves *doable,* as he chipperly introduced his plans for "very, very inexpensive small dwelling projects that would take a week or two to build." Obviously Walker had neither my proficiency nor Charlie's architecture in mind. If I strung together all the days I ended up working on it, my own first-person house took closer to six months to build and cost somewhere on the far side of $125 a square foot. (Thoreau famously claimed to have spent only $28.12½ building his cabin, but no construction cost accounting can ever be believed.) Yet, not having any way of knowing these things in advance, I began to entertain and then actually to believe that perhaps I *could* build such a building myself, and that doing so could prove not only economical and interesting but necessary in some mysterious way.

For someone as attached to words and books and chairs as I am, gratuitous physical labor wouldn't ordinarily hold much appeal. Yet I had lately developed—in the garden, as it happened—an appreciation for those forms of knowledge that seem to yield most readily to the hands. Different kinds of work, performed with different sets of tools, can disclose different faces of the world, and my work in the garden had revealed a face of nature I'd never seen before, not as a reader or a spectator. What I'd gleaned there was a taste of what the "green thumb" has in abundance, this almost bodily sense of plants and the earth that comes from handwork, sweat, and a particular quality of attention that involves very little intellect, but all of the senses. It reminded me just how much of reality slips through the net of our words, and that time spent working directly with the flesh of the world is the best antidote for abstraction.

Of course I knew something about gardening. And while it seems to me building has some striking things in common with gardening—both are ways of giving shape to a landscape; of joining elements of nature and culture to make things of usefulness and beauty; of, in effect, teasing meaning from a tree—the intellectual and physical abilities each discipline calls for could scarcely be more different. In the garden a casual approach to geometry, a penchant for improvisation, and a preference for trial and error over the following of directions will rarely get you into serious trouble. Building a house is another story. It seemed to me that the difference between gardening and building was a little like the difference between cooking (which I like to do) and baking (which I can't), a difference that has everything to do with one's attitude toward recipes. Mine has always been cavalier.

Yet after a while the sheer improbability of building something myself became the most important reason for attempting it. Just because I hadn't come by the necessary skills or habits of mind naturally (and certainly not genetically) didn't mean I couldn't cultivate them. During the renovation of our house I'd spent enough time observing the intricate discipline of the architect and wondering at the carpenter's fluency with the things of this world to have acquired an admiration for these alien habits of mind, and over time my admiration blossomed into envy. Watching the carpenters patiently translate Charlie's sheaf of abstractions into the reality of a habitable and meaningful room, I realized that what I beheld was the very foil of my own impatient and disorderly brain.

Straight and plumb, square and level, right and true: To someone like me, who can always see at least two sides of every issue, who spends his days in the company of words he dearly loves but knows better than to trust, these concepts glistened in the light of an obsolete but still longed-for certainty. Staunch, dependable, beyond the reach of argument, they were qualities you could actually build a house with. I envied all that: the deliberate, first-this-then-that of architecture, the old reliable syntax of carpentry, the raising of nonmetaphorical structures on the nonmetaphorical ground.

Writers sometimes like to draw glib parallels between building and writing, but it seemed to me nothing could be farther from the truth. Did the writer inhabit a world where "true" and "right" were things you could ascertain, where abstractions stood or fell of their own weight, where the existence of something didn't depend on a consensus? At the end of his day the builder alone could say—and yet didn't need to say, because *there it was*—he had added something to the stock of incontestable reality, created a new fact. It sounded too good to be true. This might not be a universe where I'd feel even remotely at home, but it was one that I resolved to visit, in the hope of finding something I needed to know.

≡

I was in no hurry to tell anyone about the do-it-myself part of my plan, fully expecting a cold shower of skepticism, if not outright ridicule. Judith especially, who was already armed with many excellent reasons to be dubious about the project, had to be approached carefully. As she pointed out the first time I broached the idea to her, over dinner one evening, she'd never once seen me try to repair a broken chair, let alone build anything from scratch. But I was ready for this, and the notion that I was proposing to build the thing myself *precisely because* I was so ill-equipped to do so proved to be a deft rhetorical stroke, a jujitsu move that effectively disarmed her skepticism by embracing it. By the end of the conversation Judith could fairly be described as supportive, though she strongly, and as it turned out wisely, urged that I look for someone who could help me—someone, as she put it, "who at least has a clue."

When I finally decided to call Charlie, we'd been living in the house he'd designed for nine months, and already the place fit us like a set of familiar clothes. We were almost whole again financially, and the bruises of the construction process had all but healed. For now, I was working in the loft of the barn where Judith paints, and that was tolerable—as long as I didn't mind the turpentine fumes rising from her palette in winter, the atticlike heat that collected up there in summer, and the yammering drizzle of her talk radio all year long. Painters and writers clearly use different sides of the brain when working, which makes sharing a sound system, if not a space, virtually impossible. The barn loft was a room to work in, but it certainly wasn't a room of my own.

Since moving back into the house, I'd gotten into the habit of dressing in front of the bedroom window, a fine vantage from which to assess the daily progress of the seasons, the weather, the garden. This is the window where I'd stood with Charlie a year before, and every morning I'd find myself drawn to the same spot, daydreaming my way down the garden path, a shirt button at a time, in the general direction of that notion of his, which by now seemed very much my own. I still wasn't picturing anything terribly specific, not yet. But no longer nothing, either.

And so on one of those mornings, in the spring before the summer that brought Isaac, I called Charlie first thing to tell him my plan. I told him that not only did I want to go ahead with the building we'd discussed, but that I was thinking of building it myself. I expected a protest, and probably would have backed right off had I detected any sign of one. But Charlie didn't even inhale hard. He acted as if my being a builder were the most natural thing in the world. Which was daunting.

I told him that, much as I appreciated his offer of a free design, I intended to pay him for it. But he needed to understand that whatever plan he came up with, it had to be simple enough for someone like me to build.

"You mean idiot-proof," Charlie said; he hadn't asked.

"I won't take that personally."

I launched into a rambling monologue about the little temple I envisioned. "It could be like a . . . with a desk looking out on . . . and we can't forget to . . ."—this long flight of long-pent words straining to capture this still dreamy room of my own. Charlie let me go on like this for a while. And then he broke in to ask a perfectly straightforward question to which I had no answer.

"So where do you want to put this building?"

Aside from someplace in the landscape framed by that window, I had no idea. Much as I'd been daydreaming about the building, I'd neglected to settle on a spot for it. I hadn't even ventured out those three hundred feet to walk the land yet, at least not on foot. I realized I'd flunked my first test in Concrete Reality.

"Look, there's no point talking about this or any other building in the abstract," Charlie explained, "because the site is going to dictate so much about it. This thing is one kind of guy if we perch him on the edge of the meadow looking back toward the house, and something completely different if he's sitting off in the woods all by himself. So that's the first thing you need to do . . ."

Charlie was trying, gently, to bring me and my daydreamy notion down to the ground.

First this, then that.

The time had come for me to site my building, to fix this dream of mine to the earth.

CHAPTER 2

The Site

Settling on the site of a new building is a momentous act, at least if you stop to think about it. That
not everybody does is obvious from all those buildings that crouch like strangers on their own land,
looking out of place or simply oblivious. Yet it may
be that you can think *too much* about site selection. Because deciding on the right place to build
is also uncannily simple, a process in which the
advice of the senses and intuition is often your
most reliable guide. I of course came to this realization very late, and only by the most roundabout
path.

The momentousness of the decision was *all* I
could think about. Wherever I put my building, it
would stay, more or less forever. I'd have to live

with the consequences of the choice as long as I was around, and others would be stuck with it after that. Charlie had said that key elements of my building's design, its scale and skin and fenestration, the way it met the ground and the pitch of its roof, would be determined by this first fact. Then there were the views to consider (from the building, and of the building), the fall of light across its floor, the movement of air around it, the ambient sounds, the angle at which it met the late-day sun. Dwell too long on so many soon-to-be-set-in-stone characteristics and the decision is liable to paralyze you. I know, I am only talking about a hut, an outbuilding. Yet I felt that by choosing its site—a single place out of all possible places in which to build—I was setting this great big contingency in motion, rolling it down the steep, one-way hill of personal and local history.

Faced with any such large decision, my first instinct (if you can call it that) is to look for a book to tell me what to do. But I was surprised to find that the literature of architecture and building contains remarkably little on the subject. Lewis Mumford had complained back in the fifties that the proper siting of houses was a lost art, and I turned up little to suggest it has since been found.

Mumford pointed me all the way back to Vitruvius, whose famous treatise on architecture, written in the first century B.C., offers some sensible advice on the siting of cities, dwelling houses, and tombs, all of which, he maintained, should be located according to the same principles. Vitruvius advises the prospective builder to seek a spot that is neither too high (where exposure to wind is a problem) nor too low (where it may be subject to the "poisonous breath of the creatures of the marshes"). He cautioned that a site can be intrinsically unhealthy and recommended that the builder slaughter an animal that had grazed on it and examine its liver for signs of disease. But nothing deserved closer consideration than a building site's position with respect to the sun, and Vitruvius spelled out principles of orientation that have not been improved on (which is not to say they have always been heeded): Buildings should be laid out on an east-west axis, with their principle exposure to the south. This means that in the Northern Hemisphere the low angle of the sun in winter will keep the building warm, while during the summer, when the sun passes overhead, direct sunlight will enter only in the morning and evening, when it will be welcome. For the same reason, he recommended an eastern exposure for bedrooms, western for dining rooms.

Remarkably, American architecture had to rediscover these simple rules in the 1970s, when the Arab oil embargoes suddenly made heating oil precious. For a long time before that, our houses had been plunked down pretty much anywhere a developer's lot-lines dictated. According to Mumford, Americans have never been particularly sensitive to site, a fact he attributes partly to cheap energy and partly to the eighteenth-century scheme, promoted by Thomas Jefferson, to impose a great Cartesian grid over most of the nation's land, with no regard for topography, drainage, or grading, let alone aesthetics or convenience. This division of the country into equal, square parcels of land may have made for easy surveying and speculation, but it discouraged the sensitive siting of buildings.

Of course there is more to choosing a site than orientation to the sun. For example, what sort of topography was I looking for? How should the new building relate to the house? How do you go about judging the relative hospitality of a patch of ground? What exactly was my place in this particular landscape? As far as I could tell, the Chinese had been the only culture to devise a systematic method of site selection. But fêng shui sounded very arcane to me, if not kooky, and for a long time I avoided reading anything about it. I eventually found myself turning to the garden designers, who seemed, at least in the West, to have thought more about how architecture should fit into the landscape than the architects had.

The most pertinent advice I found was in the garden literature of the eighteenth century in England, when for a brief moment, some of the best minds of the culture, from Alexander Pope to Horace Walpole to Joseph Addison, turned their attention to landscape design. These writers had thought long and hard about exactly what constituted a "pleasing prospect," as well as about the aesthetic and psychological experience of landscape, and since the picturesque gardens they promoted made abundant use of small outbuildings, which they called *follies*—a word I strove to keep as far from discussions of my project as possible—there seemed to be a lot that applied.

Since the original impetus for my building had begun with the notion of improving the view from our new bedroom window, the romantic designers—who were among the first people in the West to develop a taste for natural scenery—seemed ideally suited to the project. They worked to make every prospect in their gardens look "natural." What they meant by this was that a landscape should look not like nature as we commonly find it, and as I had found it outside my window, but as it appears in landscape paintings— "works of Nature [being] most pleasant," Addison wrote, "the more they resemble those of art." In the landscape paintings the Romantics revered, nature tends to be well-composed (divided into foreground, middle ground, and background) and pleasingly varied (particularly in terms of light and dark). It also offers the spectator's eye an inviting path to follow from one element to another, but especially from the foreground to the distant horizon.

Without being conscious of it, the dissatisfaction Judith and I had felt with the new view from our bedroom window probably owed something to our picturesque expectations, which most of us acquire growing up in this culture. All the elements of a pleasing landscape were present—fields and trees and even, now that we'd dug a small pond, water—yet there was something wrong with the picture. It was uninviting. Specifically, the scene offered the eye no reason to travel from the foreground to the background, or any path on which to do so. By adding what the Romantic designers used to call an eye-catcher, we were hoping to tie the little fortress of cultivation down by the house into the broader landscape above.

But exactly where in the picture should my eye-catcher go? My first impulse had been to put the building somewhere along an imaginary line extending out from the main axis of the garden. For many years, this line, after following the fieldstone wall and the perennial border, would pass through the arbor and then lapse into an impassable tangle of boulders and brush. This particular no-man's-land occupied the space between a pair of fine but inaccessible trees, one a white ash and the other a great, leaning white oak. The situation was somewhat improved after we dug the pond and used the spoils from the excavation to regrade the rocky area between the two trees. Today, the path journeys out to the pond, skirts its north bank, and then climbs what is now a gentle, grassy rise between the ash and the oak before settling in a small, circular meadow drawn around a stunted old swamp maple.

It seemed to me there were a couple of possible building sites along this axis, the most obvious being the bank of the pond. And for a while a pond-house seemed like an appealing idea. I could picture a little shingled shack with a dock out front jutting over the water. Though I eventually discarded this idea (it seemed too cute), it did help me appreciate how a particular site could shape my image of the building. I also rejected the site beneath the oak; the tree branched so high overhead it didn't look as though it would afford a building much sense of shelter.

But I'd also begun to doubt the wisdom of building right on the main axis of the house and garden, and in this I found strong support among the picturesque designers I consulted. They detested straight lines on aesthetic as well as political grounds—axes being closely associated with "the formal mockery of princely gardens" on the continent—and made sure their paths always curved. A path that eventually relinquished its geometry seemed in keeping with the character of this landscape, which is to grow progressively

less tended the further you travel from the house. There was also
something a little too obvious about a building that confronted you
at the end of such a straight line. Putting it on axis would make it
seem closer too, when my goal, I'd begun to realize, was to make
these few acres feel more like a world. But if instead I situated the
building at an angle to the main axis, and then made the approach
to it slightly roundabout, the workings of perspective and psychology would make it appear that much farther away—and make the
property seem that much larger.

Now I was approaching the problem as a picturesque designer
might, deploying a bit of pictorial illusion to "improve" the landscape and entice the viewer into the scene. I imagined that a
Capability Brown or William Kent would have objected to my
original plan to site the building in the sun-filled center of the
view on the grounds that it would rob the scene of mystery; better
to tuck it into a corner of the frame, preferably in a spot where it
would be partially obscured in shade. The site should be visible
from the house, they would recommend, but only just. The idea is
for it merely to catch the eye, to pique the viewer's curiosity without satisfying it. The location of an eye-catcher should make the
viewer want to venture out to the building, there to experience an
entirely different sort of mood than the one on offer near the
house.

This was no small point, for the picturesque designers were interested in much more than composing pretty pictures. They were
concerned with time and movement too, and conceived of their
landscapes in three dimensions, striving to make them work as
narratives as well as paintings. Follow the path through a picturesque landscape and you will come upon a succession of distinct places, each designed to evoke a different emotion.

I didn't have anything so fancy in mind, but I did like the idea
that the site for my building would offer a different kind of experience than the rest of the property, as well as a new perspective on

things. Of course this vastly complicated my site selection. For now I needed not only to find a spot that would add something to the view from the house, but one that would offer its own interesting views, a good place in its own right.

The time had come for me to climb down from my second-floor perch and walk the land. Apart from the turning of pages, I hadn't yet lifted a finger to bring my building any closer to reality. But thinking picturesquely had taken me some distance, narrowed my search. Now at least I knew the frame in which the site had to fit and where in that frame the site should *not* fall: the too-obvious middle. That still left a lot of ground to cover, however. I called Charlie to see if he had any advice. He did, though at the time it seemed too glib to be of much use. "Think about it this way," he suggested. "You've been hiking all day, it's getting late, and you're looking for a good campsite—just a comfortable, safe-feeling place to spend the night. That's your site."

≡

"At a certain season of our life," Thoreau wrote in *Walden,* "we are accustomed to consider every spot as the possible site of a house." Now I entered my own such season, though I didn't manage to approach it quite as lightly as Thoreau. (Of course Thoreau was never serious about settling; I was.) The first time I walked the land was a bright June afternoon, the sun directly overhead, and I quickly lost myself in my perambulations. I traced patterns across the property that would have looked antic had Judith or some neighbor happened to notice me, pacing first this way, then that, doubling and then tripling back again, before stopping to appraise a view, a deliberative process that involved a long, slow pirouette through 360 degrees. The second time out, I brought along a chair, planting it in a succession of auspicious-seeming spots, the better to rehearse inhabiting them and observe the landscape's constantly changing face.

From out here the whole problem of site selection looked somewhat different. I realized I wasn't just looking for a view, but for something more personal than that—a point of view. What would be my angle on things when I sat down to work? Some spots where I put my chair implied an oblique angle on the world, while others met it more forthrightly. I could see that I was going to have to decide whether I was a person more at home in the shadows, or out in the sunny middle of things. How important to me was the company of a tree, or the reflection of water? Just how available to the gaze of others—on the road, in the house—did I wish the face of my building to be? Some sites I considered offered what seemed like the geographical correlative of shyness, others self-assertion. It was as though the landscape were asking me to declare myself, to say this place, and not that one, suited me, in some sense *was* me.

And not just for the moment or month or year. ("And there I did live," Thoreau wrote of the sites he surveyed, "for an hour, a summer and a winter life . . .") No, this was for keeps, and there were times when I felt that choosing a site had become a metaphor for every other fateful decision I'd ever had to make, but especially all those ones that went under the decidedly un-Thoreauvian rubric of Settling Down: buying the house, signing the note, getting married, deciding to have the baby, taking the job, giving up the job. (Had Thoreau done *any* of these things?) None of these decisions had come easy, and yet it helped to remind myself that not one of them had ever given me a moment's regret either. Maybe I'm the kind of person who just needs to think all his second thoughts in advance. As Thoreau pointed out in *Walden,* there's freedom in deliberation (literally: "from freedom"); once that's over, though, things start looking a good deal more fatelike. Odd as it sounds, there were moments when I felt as though I was picking out not a building site but a cemetery plot—when I felt *that* sort of bottomless claustrophobia in time.

Which is why I took my sweet time about it, spending un-counted hours walking the property, at every time of day, in every weather, by every conceivable route. I planted my chair in two dozen places, cataloging their qualities, cataloging my responses to their qualities, until I found myself beginning to doubt, in the same way saying a word over too many times can make you doubt its sense, whether I could even say what a place was any longer, what it was that made a place a place. Was I really cataloging their qualities—shyness, forthrightness—or was I inventing them? Was a place something made, in other words, or was it something given?

"Wherever I sat, there I might live," Thoreau had written of his own less-fraught wanderings in search of a house site, "and the landscape radiated from me accordingly." And it was true that the landscape did seem to reorganize itself around me and my chair as I imagined inhabiting each site in turn. What had one moment seemed an undistinguished corner of second-growth forest, or an indifferent section of meadow grown up in goldenrod, would all of a sudden become the center of the world. My chair reminded me of the jar in the Wallace Stevens poem, an ordinary bit of human artifice that "took dominion everywhere" and ordered the "slovenly wilderness" around it. This seemed to suggest I could build just about anywhere, since anywhere I raised four corners and a roof would perforce *become* a place, almost as if by fiat. What is a place after all but a bit of space that people like me have invested with meaning?

And yet not everywhere felt equally right. Tested against Char-lie's advice, the area within the round meadow, for example, did not feel like a very comfortable place to set up camp. It was too easy to imagine eyes in the encircling trees. Also, a spot like that was always going to feel a little arbitrary. Why not pitch the tent ten feet this way, or twenty that? I might have succeeded in mak-ing a good place there, but I would be starting virtually from scratch. Perhaps my landscape, or my sense of landscape, was not as democratic as Thoreau's, or Stevens's, because certain spots proclaimed themselves more loudly to me as places *already*—the landscape seemed to radiate out from them, as it were, even before I happened to plant my seat there.

There was, for example, this one particular area—right away I want to call it a place—that seemed almost to exert a kind of gravitational pull whenever I drew near it. It was a small, unexpected clearing on the south side of a boulder easily as big as a subcompact car. I recognized the rock from one of Judith's paintings; she'd spent the better part of one summer working in this clearing. I kept returning to this spot in my wanderings, something it occurred to me my predecessor's cows had probably also once done, for the clearing opened right onto the shady path they trudged from the barn each morning on their march to the upper pasture.

The floor of the clearing, which is hidden from the cow path by the big rock, is pitched, but at a much gentler angle than the path, making it feel almost becalmed, like a small, placid eddy shunted off to the side of a rushing river. I remembered Judith mentioning what a pleasant place it had been to work. It's not hard to imagine cows stepping off the path to rest here, lying down with their broad sides to the boulder's south face, which would hold the sun's warmth when the leaves were off the trees. But they'd pause here in summer too, since the clearing then is shaded and cool. The "placeness" of this spot seemed unmistakable, even to cows.

A half-dozen young trees rise along the base of the rock, white birches and choke cherries mostly, with long flexing trunks that arc out over the clearing and open their thin canopies directly above it. Overhead, they interlace their leaves and branches with another rank of trees that lean over to meet them from the far side of the clearing, joining to form a high, almost Gothic arch. This second group of trees, which contains more cherry and birch as well as some white ash and silver maple, forms a rough hedgerow, strewn with boulders, that divides the clearing from the lower meadow. The farmer probably dug out and dragged these boulders from this field when he first plowed it, and the trees grew up among them, colonizing any spot his tractor couldn't reach. From the clearing you can peer through their silhouetted trunks into the sun-filled field.

Early one morning at the end of June I brought Judith, who was seven months pregnant, back to look over the spot, since by now it was under serious consideration as my site. As we followed the curving path I'd worn through the rough grass and weeds, I realized the route was in keeping with good picturesque practice: You registered several distinct changes in the mood of the landscape as you moved from the lucid, sun-lit geometries of the house and garden, up around the pond and into the shadowy woodland, where you even passed by a suitably melancholy ruin—a collapsed handyman's shack. When Judith stepped into the clearing, she pointed out the good light; this is what had drawn her to the place originally. The sunlight here was uncommonly delicate, finely divided by the relatively small leaves of the trees overhead, and made lively by the birch leaves, which the slightest hint of a breeze was enough to flutter.

Together we examined the views. Two of them were very fine. Looking back toward the house, the landscape sloped down in the middle distance to the pond, which was neatly framed by the big oak and ash and provided a welcome still point in the rolling scene. Beyond the pond stood the rose arbor, now clothed in deep purple clematis, and the path back to the house. It wasn't what you'd call a picturesque view, since so much in the picture looked cultivated rather than natural—"gardenesque" seemed more like it. But there was something appealing about gazing down from this shady, unseen lair onto such a sunny, well-tended scene, with its enterprising geometries of house and garden. Here was all our familiar handiwork—the clipped apple trees and the right-angled beds, the tidy stone walls and the rose climbing up the trellis on the back porch—but the new perspective, which was angled obliquely to the property's layout and elevated several degrees above it, rendered everything slightly unfamiliar.

One hundred and eighty degrees in the opposite direction offered a less tended but equally appealing view. Here was a dark funnel of foliage—the cow path—conducting your eye through the woods toward the upper pasture, where all of a sudden the green field detonated in the sun. The view reminded me of the moment at the baseball stadium when you first catch sight of the blazoned green playing field at the end of the dark alley burrowing beneath the stands.

Not all the views were quite this good, however. To the north, above the rock, it was only fifty or so yards as the crow flies to the neighbor's raised ranch, and though right now, in high summer, I couldn't see it for the trees, during the seven months of the year when the leaves are down the house's canary yellow vinyl siding would be on display. The dilapidated green cape house of another neighbor, a cranky old guy who lived alone, was also visible to the southeast, on the far side of the small meadow. His frequent tumultuous efforts to raise a wad of phlegm, the report of which rolled like thunder across the intervening meadow, offered regular reminders that this place wasn't paradise.

I stayed behind while Judith walked back toward the house; when she reached the door, I stood up on my chair waving my arms so she could get some idea of what the building might look like from the house. I shouted to her to have a look from the bedroom. She reappeared in the second-floor window, giving me the thumbs up. I sat down in my chair to take stock.

The spot certainly had a good aura about it. Whether it was the rock or the light or the clearing, you felt right away that this was somehow a privileged place. I thought of Charlie's campsite test. Except for the fact that the ground sloped a few degrees, the site seemed to meet its requirements. A tent pitched in this clearing would have the boulder to its north, providing protection from the wind and maybe even a bit of residual warmth during the night. Tucked under these trees with the big rock at your back, this did not seem like it would be a scary place to spend the night. You could see a lot from here without being easily seen yourself.

This last seemed like a particularly fitting quality for the building I had in mind. The hut was going to be my study, after all, a place in which to think and read and write—to observe the world in solitude. The site seemed to chime with my dream for the place, especially the obliqueness of its angle on things, the company of the boulder, the delicate shade—too thin for melancholy, but shadowy enough that you didn't feel exposed and not so cheerful that you couldn't think. The betweenness of the site seemed auspicious too; its sense of standing on the hedgey margin of things, between field and wood, sun and shadow. The place stood apart, and I knew it was that part of me—the self that stood a little apart—that I intended this building to house.

I moved my chair this way and that, trying to decide which direction I'd want my desk to face. The untended landscape that Thoreau would no doubt have opted for—the one looking up through the woods to the field of overgrown grasses—didn't appeal to me nearly as much as it should have. (When Charlie first saw the site, he automatically assumed the building would face the field.) It was a beautiful view, especially when the meadow's grasses burst into light at the end of the shadowy corridor. But to face that way meant turning my back on the house and garden, on that whole middle landscape Judith and I had worked so hard to make, and which I liked to write and think about. So I turned my chair 180 degrees around, positioning it so that the two big trees framed the gardens and the house, and then I took my seat there in the cool of the shade. There it was, my life, flooded in summer light, clear as day. There was the childhood home of my child-to-be, the house I was about to be the dad of. There in the open window was my wife, moving pregnantly across our bedroom. And I realized then that though I may have wanted a hut in the woods, it was definitely not Thoreau's cabin in the wilderness that I was after. It might be that I wished for a place that stood a little apart from this life of mine, but only to get a better view.

I also realized, sitting there before my imaginary desk, that the image of my hut was growing steadily more concrete. What had originally been conceived in two dimensions, a feature in a landscape as seen from a window, was now acquiring a third: I had begun to see the building from the inside out. The hut dream had a setting now; looking out at the world through its imaginary windows, I felt reasonably sure this was it.

=

By now there should have been no question that this was indeed the place. All the picturesque angles checked out, it'd passed Charlie's campsite test, I thought I'd felt its gravitational pull. I've never been a great one for trusting my instincts, however. And though I liked the view quite a lot, surely there were a dozen other potential sites with a similar orientation. What did it really mean, anyway, to say a "place felt right," or that it had a "good aura"? It all was starting to sound a little New Age—y to me.

You see, I was having another instinct, which was to find an intellectual theory to second my first instinct. That's why I'd looked up the picturesque landscape designers in the first place. But now I wondered if I couldn't find an entirely different theory to confirm me in my choice or, failing that, point me toward another.

The time had come to read a few books about fêng shui. This was a chore I'd been putting off since a couple of years before when I'd picked up a treatise on the subject in a bookstore and came upon the following sentence: "The greatest generation of chi occurs at the point where the loins of the dragon and the tiger are locked together in intercourse." What exactly do you do with a tip like that? A line drawing sought to clarify the point: It showed a dragon superimposed over one ridge of mountains confronting a tiger superimposed on a second ridge; in between them, down where their midsections met, an X marked the optimal site for your house or tomb. (There it was again!) I really couldn't see how such an approach could possibly help me, but I decided to try.

The first fêng shui primer I consulted—*The Living Earth Manual of Feng-Shui* by Stephen Skinner—said that "the amount of chi flowing, and whether it accumulates or is rapidly dispersed at any particular point, is the crux of fêng shui." "Chi" is the Chinese word for the earth spirit, or cosmic breath, which flows in invisible (but predictable) currents over the face of the earth, following both the natural and manmade contours of the landscape. This earth spirit animates all living things, and the more of it that enters and lingers in your building, the better. Though matters soon get more complicated, the basic objective seemed to be to find a site well supplied with chi.

I found it helpful to think of fêng shui as the terrestrial counterpart of astrology. It is concerned with the influence of the earth spirit on human life in much the same way that astrology is concerned with the influence of the heavenly bodies. But while there's nothing we can do to influence the planets' paths, there is apparently a great deal we can do to influence the path of chi through a landscape, first through proper site selection and then through site improvement. In this respect fêng shui is a form of gardening. Like picturesque garden theory, it tells you how to improve a landscape, but to spiritual rather than aesthetic ends.

So where do the dragons and tigers come in? Evidently the Chinese visualize the tallest forms in a landscape as a writhing dragon, and this high ground is the wellspring of chi. "The ridges and lines in the landscape form the body, veins, and pulse of the dragon," Skinner writes, and the dragon's "veins and watercourses [known as dragon lines] both carry the chi" down from the highest elevations. (You might assume that maximum quantities of chi will be found at the top of a hill, which is true, but because exposure to the four winds disperses chi so quickly, hilltops are generally considered poor sites.) The tiger is a similar though less prominent land form. A good site will have a dragon to its east and a tiger to its west, and face south, which the Chinese regard as the most beneficent of the cardinal points. Stripped of animal metaphors, the practical import of this principle is that people should build among hills, on ground neither too high nor too low, on a site that is open to the south and has higher ground to its north—advice, by the way, that Vitruvius would enthusiastically endorse. A more general rule of fêng shui holds that the topography of a site should strike a balance between yang land forms (the "male" ones, which tend to be upright) and flatter yin, or female, ones, such as plains or bodies of water.

My brain crammed with these elementary principles, I paid a visit to the site, aiming to see it now with the eye of the geomancer, or fêng shui doctor. It appeared I had a good balance of yin and yang, since the site stood at the meeting place of forest and field. Also, the big rock seemed to offer a suitable yang to the yin of the clearing. The land rises precipitously to the east of the site, so I had what seemed like a nice-size dragon exactly where I wanted it. But try as I might, I could not find a tiger anywhere, which was discouraging, at least until I read in one of the books that wherever you find a dragon, there will automatically be a tiger too. I had no idea how they could be so sure, but decided not to worry about it for the time being. Because right now I had chi flows to worry about.

As far as I could tell, chi has a lot in common with water. At least it helps to think of it that way, especially if your spiritual development is as retarded as mine. Like water (which also animates life), chi flows down from high ground through rills and swales in the land and then accumulates in lakes and rivers or, less propitiously, in swamps (where, hemmed in, it's apt to turn into *sha*, the negative energy that is chi's evil twin). And in fact several authorities state explicitly that water is a "conductor" of chi.

As soon as I'd begun to think of chi as flowing water, I could visualize its movement over my land, as it searched out grooves in the earth and openings in the forest on its course down the hillside. To map a landscape's dragon lines, a fêng shui doctor will sometimes travel to the top of a ridge and then run down it several times as heedlessly as possible, noting the various paths he naturally inclines toward, the points at which they intersect, and the places where his momentum is checked by hollows or inclines. The practitioner is said to be "riding the dragon," something animals do as a matter of course. (And in fact animal paths are considered reliable conduits of chi.) Though I wasn't quite prepared to ride the dragon, I thought I could picture where it would take me more or less, and it looked as though there was a positively torrential flow of chi coming down the hillside, most of it streaming down the cow path toward the pond.

This seemed auspicious. At least until I delved deeper into the literature of fêng shui and learned that the quantity of chi isn't everything—speed is just as important. And when a dragon line is particularly straight or steep, the chi is apt to travel too swiftly through the site to confer its benefits. Ideally, chi should meander through a site; torrents were no good. I felt proficient enough at visualizing the flow of chi to see that it was moving at a very rapid clip through the property, and probably whizzing right by my site in a feckless blur.

I don't mean to make fêng shui sound like a lot of hocus-pocus, because the more I learned about it, the more its images of energy flow and velocity began to square with my own more secular experience of landscape. Don't we also think of landscapes in terms of speed and energy? We commonly describe a hill as rising "slowly" or "rapidly," and we conceive of curves and straightaways in terms of their velocity. Once I began to think of fêng shui as a set of time-tested metaphors to describe a landscape, rather than as spiritual dogma, it became a lot less strange, and potentially even useful.

I realized, for example, that everything that had been done to improve our property in the last century or so—the scooping out of plateaus for the house and barn, the opening of fields on the gentler hillside slopes, the repair of the drainage around the house, and, most recently, my digging of a pond—had the unintended effect of improving the fêng shui. My predecessors here and I have been unconsciously engaged in the work of moderating what had been (and to some extent still is) a tumultuous flow of chi through the property, creating fields and ponds, plateaus and gardens where it might slow and linger, and rerouting one main artery so that it would circle around the house.

I started to see how a fêng shui doctor analyzing a given landscape's chi and the picturesque designer studying its genius loci would end up recommending much the same improvements. Both would advise that straight paths be made to curve, that flat land (where chi is thought to stagnate) be rendered more hilly and rugged ground made to slope more gently. It seemed to me that the "eye" whose attention Humphry Repton or Capability Brown spoke of attracting and directing with their clearings and paths and follies isn't so very different from the chi that fêng shui seeks to attract and direct. Likewise, the picturesque sensibility's preference for variety in the landscape—its emphasis on the transitions between field and wood, hill and dale, light and shade—might just be another way of expressing the geomancer's preference for those places in the landscape where yin and yang land forms meet. I don't know if it's ever been checked out, but I would bet that the fêng shui of English landscape gardens is exemplary.

Over the years my own landscape had come a long way, in fêng shui as well as picturesque terms, though clearly there were still problems. But I figured I was better off with an oversupply of chi close by my site than a shortage of it. The question was whether it could be encouraged to stick around long enough to be of some value. And there seemed to be only one way to find out. What I attempted now was so alien to my constitution, so ridiculous to my accustomed way of thinking, that I still can't fully believe I actually did it. I told no one, not even Judith. But I decided to ride the dragon.

On the appointed afternoon I walked all the way to the top of the hillside, keeping an eye on the road to make sure I wouldn't be observed. Then I started walking fairly rapidly in the direction of my site, quickly picking up speed until I was just about flying down the hillside. I tried as best I could not to steer, emptying my mind of any specific destination. I found my feet were quickly drawn to the cow path—obviously a dragon line. And if I stayed on this course, a powerful sensation of momentum promised to propel me straight past the big rock and smack into the middle of the pond. Had I kept to that trajectory I'm not at all sure it would have been possible to stop. But when instead I leaned my weight just slightly to the left immediately before reaching the rock, something that the lay of the land seemed to encourage, I moved into the site itself and immediately felt the gentler slope of the terrain slowing my velocity, welcoming me. My body still registered some forward momentum, but now it was an easy matter to slow and pause and rest. I felt the truth of a metaphor I'd earlier used to describe the site, that of an eddy shunted off to the side of a rushing river; there was definitely an eddying of chi taking place here.

As I stood in the clearing catching my breath, it occurred to me that this episode represented the first physical effort I'd applied to the project, and it had yielded more than I would have guessed. By riding the dragon, and temporarily shelving my usual cerebrations, I'd managed to elicit the testimony of my senses, acquired a kind of bodily knowledge of my site. For though my well-read eye had prepared me to see that the clearing's fêng shui probably had a lot going for it, it was my legs that had confirmed me in this, given me a vivid, physical sense of its hospitableness. Now I knew I had— because I'd felt it—an ample, if still slightly obstreperous, supply of chi. Knew it, in fact, in my bones.

≡

But was I prepared to credit that bodily knowledge? Of course not. Reverting to type, I decided to subject my site to one last, impeccably Western test—a scientific analysis. I read up on human habitat selection, a relatively new discipline that seeks to combine the insights of sociobiology, geography, and what is called environmental psychology. I figured that if I could now justify my choice of site on scientific grounds, I'd be set.

The theory of human habitation selection was first proposed in 1975 by an English geographer named Jay Appleton and seconded, more or less, by sociobiologist E. O. Wilson in his 1984 book, *Biophilia*. The premise of this Darwinian theory seems reasonable enough: Human beings, like other animals, have a genetic predisposition to seek out for their habitats those landscapes that are most conducive to their well-being and survival. Having spent 99 percent of our time on earth as hunter-gatherers, Homo sapiens should have acquired a predilection for landscapes that offer a high degree of what Appleton calls "prospect" and "refuge": places that offer good views—of potential supplies of food as well as sources of danger—without compromising a sense of shelter. For the hunter-gatherer, those places that allow one to see without being seen have an obvious survival value.

It is no coincidence that the type of landscape richest in opportunities for prospect and refuge is the savanna, where it is thought that the species evolved. For an upright, ground-dwelling biped, these flat or gently rolling grassy plains, punctuated by bodies of water and copses of trees, are at once abundant in visible sources of food and water and relatively safe: From the shade of the trees, one can look out over a great expanse of land with little risk of detection. Sociobiologists like Wilson suggest that a predisposition toward our optimum primordial habitat survives in the form of a pronounced aesthetic preference for savanna-like landscapes—evident in the design of our parks, picturesque gardens, and suburbs.

In his collection of lectures *The Symbolism of Habitat*, Appleton demonstrates the importance of symbols of prospect and refuge in the history of landscape painting and architecture. A pleasing landscape painting or garden, he maintains, will be one that offers both kinds of symbols, along with some visual means of traveling from one to the other. Among the symbols of refuge he mentions are trees, copses, caves, and buildings; horizons, hills, and towers function as symbols of prospect, and paths or roads serve to link the two kinds of imagery, facilitating the viewer's exploration of the scene. The picturesque painters and landscape designers were masters of the symbolism of habitat, Appleton contends, and this is why their ideas and creations have endured.

Whether our attraction for the symbolism of habitat is a matter of biology or simply an old and successful habit, Appleton's theory does help account for the gravitational attraction we feel toward certain kinds of landscapes—and, specifically, for the attraction I felt for my site. For certainly the clearing by the rock offered a high degree of prospect and refuge. Any rock this big affords a sense of refuge, and this particular rock—at the wooded edge of a field, and overlooking a pond—offered fine prospects as well. On my next visit to the site, I decided to try to see it through Paleolithic eyes. The perspective of a twentieth-century hunter was the best I could manage, but I could easily imagine such a person crouched down close to the rock, peering unseen into the lower field or down toward the pond, where grazing animals would be apt to congregate. Prospect and refuge, seeing without being seen: this was the very essence of my site.

So could it be my site had the sanction of the human genome itself? Maybe my instinct about the place (my first instinct, that is, not the subsequent one that drove me into the stacks) was the voice of some dim primordial urge—maybe, in other words, it was not merely a metaphorical instinct but the actual genetic mechanism that governs human habitat selection. It's hard for me to think of myself as being even remotely in touch with such a thing (hence instinct number two). But perhaps this is where Charlie's campsite test comes in: The exercise of trying to imagine a place as a safe spot to sleep is a way of putting us in closer touch with any deep, atavistic impulses we might feel about it. For what is camping, after all, but a temporary reversion to the life of the hunter-gatherer? Sleeping outdoors, beyond the envelope of civilization and technology, instantly renders the value of prospect and refuge vivid once again.

At first it seemed uncanny to me that the three different perspectives I'd tried out on my site could have overlapped so closely. Yet of course if the scientific perspective is correct, and there is some biological basis for our landscape preferences, we should probably not be too surprised that cultures as different from one another as Ming Dynasty China and Augustan England would have developed vocabularies that find so many similar things to praise in a landscape: Both may be articulating the same deep attractions.

Yet what confirmed me in my choice finally was no one test, but the very fact that all three perspectives—science and art and mysticism—had evidently concurred: this uncanny, almost mystical alignment of theories and metaphors. The analysis to which I subjected my site may have had all the trappings of rational inquiry, and I suppose I brought the proper enlightenment skepticism to bear on the process, but in the end what was I really doing? Hunting for a patch of sacred ground on which to build, and an authority—or, in my case, three authorities—to consecrate it, to say, Yes, this clearing in the woods is the right place.

I figured that if the artist, the geomancer, and the scientist all agree, then maybe this place was really as special as it felt. None of them may possess the "truth" about what makes a good site, but together they represent a couple thousand years of human experience of the land, which might be as close to the truth of the matter as I could hope to get.

It's possible that this almost magical sense of place I've been describing is an anachronism, something we will overcome as we accustom ourselves to the Enlightenment idea of space that Thomas Jefferson was advancing with his great grid—the powerful concept that space is the same everywhere, that it's continuous, centerless, edgeless, and organized in strict adherence to the laws of Euclidean geometry. Someday we may feel perfectly at home on the big Cartesian grid, giving our addresses in x, y, and z coordinates.

And yet powerful as this notion of space is, I've discovered it doesn't rhyme very well with the body's own experience of space, whether riding the dragon or simply sitting in a chair. The testimony of our senses seems adamant that space is full of interruptions and breaks and places qualitatively different one from another—places that seem to us special, if not magical. All the vocabularies of place I consulted, and the long human experience they represent, concur in the conviction that space is in fact discontinuous, that place is sometimes found and not made—that there is finally something more than a modernist's glass jar giving structure to the landscape. Something like these bodies of ours.

That jar of Wallace Stevens's notwithstanding, ever since the day I stumbled on this site it has felt like a place I found rather than chose. Sitting out here on a summer afternoon in this sweet, sweet spot of shade, raising up around me these four imaginary walls and perfecting in imaginary rafters the roof of arching boughs that partially shelters me already, the sense that here is a good place to be, to build, seems a fact fully as real, as given, as the big rock sitting here beside me. How could I ever have doubted it? I may have come to this knowledge the long way around, but now I understood—*knew in my bones!*—what the farmer's dumbest cow had understood without a moment's bovine reflection. This is the place.

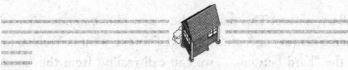

CHAPTER 3

On Paper

1. WORDS

By now you have probably noticed a tendency of mine to lean rather heavily on words and theories in my dealings with the world. How else to account for my inability to pick a spot for a building without recourse to a half-dozen books and three different theories of site selection? And yet it was partly in order to get away from words that I was attracted to the idea of building something with my own hands in the first place.

"Information overload" is something we hear a lot about these days, and there does seem to be a growing sense that technology, the media, and the sheer quantity of information in circulation have somehow gotten between us and reality—what used to be called, without a lot of quotation marks or qualifiers, nature. This may not be a new phenomenon—it was more than a century ago, after all, that Thoreau went to Walden to recover the "hard bottom . . . we can call reality" from the "mud and slush of opinion" that obscured it—but the situation does seem to have gotten worse. Not only is the mud and slush of opinion a lot thicker now that it's being piled on by so many different media, but our most famous philosophers (think of Jacques Derrida or Richard Rorty) are telling us that, underneath it all, there may not be any reality to recover—that it's mud and slush all the way down.

I suffer from an acute case of the contemporary malady, one that probably goes back to a time before people had coined terms like "information overload" and "media saturation" or thought to attach the word "virtual" to "reality." I remember as a teenager reading that Marshall McLuhan had likened opening the Sunday paper to settling into a warm bath. The metaphor delivered a tiny jolt of recognition, because I too found reading—reading almost anything—to be a vaguely sensual, slightly indulgent pleasure, and one that had very little to do with the acquisition of information. Rather than a means to an end, the deep piles of words on the page comprised for me a kind of soothing environment, a plush cushion into which sometimes I could barely wait to sink my head. More often than not, I could remember almost nothing the moment I lifted myself out of the newspaper or magazine or paperback in which I'd been immersed. Not that I usually bothered to try. Mostly I just let the print wash over me, as if it were indeed warm water, destined to swirl down the drain of my forgetfulness.

So it's probably not surprising that I should have grown up to be a magazine editor and a writer, someone who might reasonably be described as a professional producer of bathwater for others. But even after long days spent editing copy or writing, I never go anywhere without packing something to read. I'm pained to be caught on the subway without a book or a periodical, and if by accident I should find myself in so naked a state, I'll commence reading over my seatmate's shoulder—newspapers, potboilers, bibles swaddled in plastic slipcovers—or I'll study the back pages of the tabloids arrayed in front of me, a less-than-perfect medium that nevertheless has been the source of most of what I know about sports. I'll read just about anything, in fact, before I'd even think to glance at the face of the person seated across the car or otherwise engage the parade of humanity before me.

I'm afraid it doesn't stop there. It's all I can do to resist the urge to steal a few paragraphs while I'm in the car, pumping gas, or walking down the street (three challenges I've met), and even when I'm in social or intimate situations where reading is unquestionably a poor idea. More than once, Judith has caught me as my eyes reached for a line of print right in the middle of a big heart-to-heart.

You can see why I might start to think this was a problem. I began to suspect that the gorgeous columns of words had indeed become a kind of cushion between me and the unwritten world, even a crutch. And then, a few years ago, the tiny voice whispering that I might be missing something spending so much of my time in the tub was amplified by a sentence I read (on the subway, as it happened) in a book by Hannah Arendt, a sentence that kept coming back to me as a kind of rebuke. "Nothing perhaps is more surprising in this world of ours," the philosopher wrote, "than the almost infinite diversity of its appearances, the sheer entertainment value of its views, sounds, and smells, something that is hardly ever mentioned by the thinkers and philosophers." At first, this sentence struck me as being poignant, even profound. But then, with this piercing sense of deflation, I realized that anybody who regarded this observation as anything but obvious—as anything but *pathetically* obvious—had a serious problem.

And that included me. To make matters worse, I didn't have the excuse of being a thinker or a philosopher to fall back on. I was just a magazine editor, a mid-level producer and consumer of bathwater who spent most of his working days neck-deep not only in "the mud and slush of opinion" but in information and statistics, images and arguments, even in *opinions* about opinion—meta–mud and slush, you could say. So perhaps it was inevitable that sooner or later the prospect of doing something more directly involved with the "views, sounds, and smells" of this world would become attractive to me, if not a matter of some therapeutic urgency. Plato, who was of course famously distrustful of all worldly appearances, wrote that in order to open the eyes of the mind we first had to close the eyes of the body. I wanted to go some distance the other way, hoping by a spell of unfamiliar and worldly work to open the eyes of the body, if only by a squinty crack.

Anyone who works with words and symbols every day will know what I'm talking about—it is the same impulse that fills the streams with anglers every April, the nurseries with gardeners, and the hardware stores with do-it-yourself carpenters. Though it turns out the matter is never quite that simple. Because no sooner have you declared your allegiance to some corner of the physical world than you discover a long, alluring shelfful of relevant books and periodicals, word upon word of irresistible how-to that it is suddenly imperative to consult. I confess that part of the appeal for me of first gardening and then carpentry were the vast new uncharted realms of print—the countless books and periodicals and mail-order catalogs—these pastimes opened up for my delectation. It is not easy, getting past words.

Yet that is what I felt a growing desire to do, and what attracted me to making a building in particular. For building seemed to me to be one of the most tangible, and grounded, and factual things that human beings do—the closest we ever come to making something on the order of nature, something with the sheer, incontrovertible presence of a tree or a rock. Instead of turning away from "worldly appearances," I would see if I couldn't make one of them myself. The work of building seemed to hold out the promise of at least a partial cure for my addiction to print, for this sense of living at too great a remove from the things of this world and the life of the senses. As it turned out I wasn't entirely wrong about this, though I was more than a little naïve.

≡

The process of designing my building began with more words, however. The best way I could think of to convey my dream for the place to Charlie was in writing. So a few weeks after I had settled on the site, I wrote him a long letter outlining what I thought my needs were and describing as best I could the building taking shape in my head. The words in this letter, along with all the other words we exchanged in the weeks to come, comprised an informal version of what architects call the program: the list of requirements and wishes that motivates any architectural undertaking. In the simplest terms, the task before Charlie was to design a form— a building—that would mediate between the desires set forth in my words on the one hand, and the facts of the site on the other.

My experience of the site, sitting out there on my chair, approaching the place time and again and considering its prospects, had deepened my sense of the building I wanted. It had begun as a simple, two-dimensional picture, something to improve a view, but by now the image of the building in my mind's eye had acquired an interior and its own point of view, and it was this that I tried to describe in my letter. There was now a long desk at one end of a rectangular room that faced in the direction of the house, taking in the pond between the trees, the garden, and the path back to the porch. Above the desk I pictured a big window. Visible from the house, this wall would constitute the building's most public face, though I pictured the door going on the opposite wall, where it wouldn't interfere with the desk; putting it on the back wall would also force you to walk around the big rock before entering the building, which seemed like a good way to approach it.

Sitting there at my imaginary desk, mentally swiveling around in my chair, I considered what else I wanted in the room. Plenty of bookshelves. A stove of some kind. A place for Judith to sit. Also high on the list was a daybed—a cozy spot to read or snooze. But how do you make a cozy spot in a one-room hut? I pictured the daybed carved into a thick wall, a niche enveloped by bookshelves or cabinets. My image here probably came from Monticello, which I'd recently visited. Jefferson sandwiched his bed in between two rooms, so that it forms a deep, snug pocket in the wall, which he could enter from either side. I had only one room to work with here—this had to be a simple building, I stressed to Charlie, if I was going to build it myself. (The word "simplicity" appears several times in the letter, usually underlined.) But what if we made one of the walls abnormally thick? The depth of a bookcase, say. This would give us a space the daybed could be fitted into, creating at least a partial sense of enclosure. A thick wall or two would also provide plenty of spaces to hold my books and other things. Part of my image of this place was that it would be meticulously organized, with everything I required built in or easily stowed—"boat-like," is how I put it in the letter to Charlie. There was no question that my streamlined new workspace was conceived under the sign of Getting Organized.

"I picture a space no bigger than it has to be," I wrote in the letter, "single in purpose and shipshape, with a specific, dedicated place for everything. We should think of the interior less as a room, in fact, than as a piece of furniture, or maybe a cockpit." I emphasized that the wall unit needn't be fancy—that it might even be part of the building's frame, use its plywood sheathing for its back. Thick walls would also serve to warm up the room, it seemed to me, by creating an intermediate space, a kind of buffer, between the inside and the outside of the building. This might make the place feel somewhat less exposed than you would expect a hut set out in the woods to feel, give it a stronger sense of refuge.

Yet there was something a little odd about this wish for thick walls, because at the same time I entertained what seemed like a completely contradictory image of the building as a place radically open to the landscape—as a room that, by virtue of its size and site, could be on far more intimate terms with nature than the house was. I asked Charlie for lots of operable windows—at least one on each wall—and even a small porch or deck where I might sit outside and read when it got too warm indoors. I guess I had very different winter and summer images of the place. Charlie would have to sort this out.

Outside, I pictured wood shingles instead of the crisp clapboards that clad the house; shingles seemed better suited to the wooded site and suggested a softer, shaggier, and generally more inviting building. And in spite of some of the fairly complicated elements I'd asked for inside, my letter emphasized that the look of the building from the outside should be plain and unselfconscious, "more chicken coop than atelier." Then, in what would prove to be an unanswered prayer, I suggested a very rough budget and invoked the principle of simplicity one last time ("remember: something an idiot can build") before dropping the letter in the mail.

I had no idea what Charlie would make of it. On one level, the letter seemed to describe a plausible-sounding place; a novelist could probably construct a coherent fictional room out of the words in my letter. But a carpenter? I wasn't so sure. The letter contained several fairly precise images of the building, yet they were all unconnected, just bits and pieces: Here was a corner with a tiny woodstove and a stuffed chair pulled up to it; over there, on one side of the desk, a small window completely filled with the face of the big rock. Then here—*some*where—was this thick wall of bookcases that was going to organize my life, like a second brain. And over there was the daybed, from which I wanted to look out on the meadow and yet at the same time feel perfectly snug. I might be able to write a logical transition from one image to the next, but could anybody begin to draw it?

Just for the hell of it, I decided to try. I drew a rectangle and started filling it up with all the different elements I'd mentioned: the desk, the daybed, the stove, the thick wall, the door, the various windows, and, hanging somewhere off of the rectangle, the porch. Very soon I ran out of walls and corners, and had begun to add on more rectangles, even to contemplate a second story. I had drawn what amounted to a pile-up of architectural notions loosely contained by a couple of rectangles; I couldn't even begin to picture what the exterior of such a structure would look like. Like my letter, my drawing was little more than a collage made up of wishes and remembered places, pictures I'd seen and things I'd read. The letter at least had a bit of syntax to keep it from flying apart.

How would an architect go about turning these words into a building? The question began to intrigue me, so when I phoned Charlie to alert him to the letter, I asked if he would be willing to let me somehow observe the process—talk to him about it along the way, and maybe even drive up to Boston to watch him draw. At first Charlie sounded game. But a few moments later, after I'd tried to engage him in a discussion of some theoretical issue in architecture I'd been reading about, he seemed to pull back. Charlie cautioned that watching him design my building wasn't necessarily going to give me a fair picture of contemporary architecture, if that's what I was looking for. "Just as long as you realize that what I do doesn't have too much to do with all that stuff."

I *hadn't* realized that, actually. Charlie had studied under a number of eminent contemporary architects—Charles Moore, at UCLA, where he went to architecture school in the late seventies; and Peter Eisenman, at the Institute for Architecture and Urban Design in New York—and his father, a former head of the architecture department at MIT, was himself fairly well known for several arresting modernist buildings in and around Boston. So Charlie wasn't exactly an architectural naïf.

I heard nothing from Charlie for a couple of weeks, and had begun to wonder what was going on when two equally perplexing items arrived in the mail. The first was a computerized notice from the magazine *Progressive Architecture* informing me that Charles R. Myer had taken out a gift subscription in my name. The second was a hand-bound booklet of photocopied photographs and drawings that Charlie had put together, with thick cardboard covers and a spiral binding. No note accompanied the booklet, and its pages were completely wordless. So here was Charlie's answer to my letter.

I flipped through it with a deepening sense of bafflement that eventually ripened into frustration. The first couple of pages weren't too bad. Here on the first spread was a collage of tiny houses, which made me think the book was probably a collection of references for the design of my studio. One of them, a tall and narrow shack set out under a bare tree in the snow, I recognized from *Tiny Houses,* and it had something of the feeling I associated with my hut and its site. The one next to it seemed way off the mark, though, a stone building with a beefy chimney and the sort of steeply pitched alpine roof I associate with some of the sounder houses in the Brothers Grimm. The second page was a site plan of our property, showing the pond and the rock in relation to the house and the axis of the garden.

But by the time I got to the third page I had started to feel lost. Here was a blueprint of the plan for a huge and bizarre-looking house consisting of three parallel axes crossed perpendicularly by a fourth. Peculiar as that drawing was, it was at least recognizable as architecture, which could not be said about what followed. On the next few pages were photocopies of a minutely detailed instruction manual for the assembly of some elaborate machine— the kind of headache-producing fig. 1 / fig. 2 diagrams that might come with a particularly intricate model airplane. Then came a page depicting several hand tools. So this section was something about an assembly kit. Maybe Charlie was trying to warn me against attempting to build the house myself?

On the next few pages were a series of drawings having to do with the Golden Section, the famous mystical proportion I'd managed in a long education to avoid learning anything about. The first drawing—of a rectangle placed inside a circle so that its long side lined up along the circle's diameter—purported to illustrate the geometry of the Golden Section and the Fibonacci Series, a sequence of numbers that evidently has something to do with it. The drawings that followed demonstrated how the same 1:1.618 ratio pops up all over the place in architecture and nature: in the elevation of the Parthenon and the wings of a butterfly; in the façade of Notre-Dame and the spiral of a seashell. Frankly I've never been sure whether to file the marvels of the Golden Section under Profound Truths of the Universe or Pot-Smokers' Koans. Now at least I knew where Charlie stood on the question. But what did it have to do with my building?

The next several pages seemed to offer a return to Planet Earth, with a series of photographs of buildings and architectural details drawn from a bewilderingly wide range of places, styles, and periods. There was a broken-down tobacco barn with airy matchstick walls; a Voysey mansion with immense chimneys and delicate fenestration; a miniature bungalow that had sprouted a small, glazed room directly above its front porch; an Old World townhouse with a whimsical façade that resembled a cat; a lattice wall grown over with a riot of vines; a massive stone house with extremely deep-seated windows; a pair of wicker rockers sitting in a room that had a thatched roof but no walls (this was one of a series of progressively odder roofs and ceilings, including one that looked like the hull of an overturned boat); a window seat cut into a deep bookcase in a sleek postmodern living room that was trimmed with

oversized columns, capitals, and a pediment; and then a complicated little room, outfitted with a built-in bed and a desk and a
wing chair, that reminded me of a sleeping compartment on a
train.

Each image was more beautiful and strange than the last; many
of them strongly evoked particular senses of place or light or texture. But what did they *mean*? I don't know if this had been Charlie's intention, but his book left me feeling as though I'd been
stranded in a place where I didn't speak the language. Though in
some of the pictures I could discern the ghostly traces of things I'd
talked about in my letter (thick and thin walls, daybeds, casement
windows), with most of them I failed to see the point. I thirsted for
captions, just a word or two to help me see what in the world a
stone mansion in England had to do with my one-room shack in
the Connecticut woods. I closed the book feeling more than a little annoyed, in fact, a feeling that only intensified after I took a
moment to study the cover design, which I'd somehow managed to
overlook before. But Charlie had made an abstract design out of
some thin slivers of balsa wood that he'd pasted to the cardboard
cover. It consisted of two parallel bars, about an inch thick and set
an inch apart, joined together by a dozen perpendicular match-
sticks, like so:

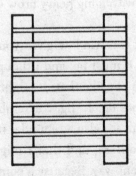

I had no idea what this was supposed to mean (if anything). Like
everything else about the book, it seemed insiderish, coy. All I

could think about was whether or not all the time Charlie'd spent putting this thing together was going to show up on my bill.

I called Charlie, hoping to find out what I was supposed to make of the booklet and to thank him for the subscription to *Progressive Architecture*. I confessed my bewilderment (the irritation I kept to myself) and asked him exactly how the book fit into the process. Charlie cheerfully explained that he'd collected these images after reading my letter, that this was something he often did at the beginning of a job. "Next time we meet, we'll go through it together. That'll give me a better sense of what's important to you, what sort of feeling you want here. I find it's usually better to hear somebody's gut reaction to a specific picture than for either of us to try to describe some sort of effect, which can get pretty abstract, and lead to misunderstandings." Charlie distrusted words, I realized; the booklet was his pointed response to my wordy and, probably to him, overly abstract letter.

I told him that I'd actually found his book kind of abstract, and couldn't always see the relevance of a particular picture to the project at hand. For instance, what was the story with that mansion?

"Isn't that guy great? I love how that bay window curves outward without ever extending beyond the wall—it's tucked in there almost like this eyeball with a big heavy brow over it."

"So?"

"Well, the curve of the window gives you a sense of just how thick the wall around it must be, and I thought maybe we want to tuck the daybed into a bay like that. It might be really neat."

And what about those fig. 1 / fig. 2 assembly instructions?

"Just a little joke. But it's also a reminder to me to keep the construction fairly simple here, and that I might want to draw this project in some different way. Because a conventional plan and elevation isn't going to tell you how all the parts fit together, or what order you need to do things in. These are things you can usually count on the contractor to figure out. But you may need something more like one of these diagrams—an instruction manual."

We arranged a time for me to come to Boston, and I thanked him for the magazine subscription. "I should warn you," Charlie said, "*PA* can get pretty wild. But you've got to read it if you want to know what's going on in architecture right now." I asked Charlie if he was a subscriber. He said he used to read it religiously but hadn't in the last couple of years. "It's a lot of fun, but I don't have time for that stuff these days. You'll see. It's not the real world."

≡

The first issue of *Progressive Architecture* to arrive happened to be its annual awards edition, its thirty-ninth, which singled out a dozen or so new projects—houses, museums, office buildings, artists' lofts—for praise.* The magazine was oversized and lavishly produced, with lots of full-color photographs on heavily coated stock. It had the look and heft and even some of the glamour of a fashion magazine. Except that all the models here were buildings—there were virtually no people in sight.

I saw right away what Charlie had meant when he said, "It's not the real world." Almost all of the award-winners were *not* real buildings—they were drawings and models of buildings that, in many cases, would never get built. This seemed peculiar. Wasn't reviewing a set of architectural drawings a little like trying to review a play without going to see it? How could you tell whether or not the building really worked before it was built? Of course I never asked this question of Charlie or anybody else; I figured it was probably naïve, and liable to mark me as unsophisticated. (Though I was amused to see a few years later that *Progressive Ar-*

---

*Progressive Architecture ceased publication in 1995, after being sold to *Architecture* magazine, which was relaunched in 2006 as *Architect*. The awards program lives on through it all, appearing each year in an issue of *Architect*.

chitecture had instituted a new department called the "post-occupancy critique," in which a reporter actually visited a building in use to see how well it worked and what the people who worked or lived there actually thought about it. This was regarded in architecture-criticism circles as a radical innovation.)

Most of the prize-winning buildings, or designs, struck me as willfully idiosyncratic and, at least before I read the lengthy captions, totally perplexing. Here was a trio of silver plywood structures on a beach, each resembling a different fish washed up on shore: a carp, a ray, and a sea slug. Called Beached Houses, they were intended as artists' housing in Jamaica. A prospective Tokyo office building designed by Peter Eisenman looked like a conventional glass-walled tower that had somehow been folded over and over again until it resembled an origami construction—a dizzying collage of multiplying facets and peculiar angles. The California architect Frank Gehry had two winners, both of them actually destined to get built. Another California architect had designed a house and gallery for an art collector in Santa Fe that consisted of two groupings of cubes within cubes within cubes; it looked like the sort of building you might get if you asked M. C. Escher to design your house. But probably the very weirdest house to win a prize wasn't even one you could look at in a model or drawing. That's because the architect proposed to *improvise* its design, so there could be no plan or elevation in advance. Periodically he planned to visit the site, look at whatever the builder had done that day and, taking his inspiration from that, make some new drawings for the next stage of construction. I guessed this was a joke on Goethe's famous aphorism likening architecture to frozen music. Here was frozen jazz.

I got the feeling there were a lot of jokes being made, and the best ones were probably sailing over my head, since they were aimed primarily at other architects and architecture critics. I seriously doubt Peter Eisenman chuckled about origami when he presented his office building scheme to his Japanese patrons. Or that the designer of the carp, ray, and sea slug in Jamaica mentioned to his client that the decision to base these artists' houses on fishes was meant as a postmodernist statement about the arbitrariness of the relationship between form and content in architecture. (Fish is to artist as form is to content?) I certainly wouldn't have known this about the project unless I'd been told.

And told we were, over and over again—in the captions, in the quotations from the architects' statements of purpose, and in the jurors' comments, which were informative and often highly entertaining. A good thing, too, because without the words, these buildings were incomprehensible indeed—sort of like Charlie's booklet, but without any of the sensual rewards.

Lewis Mumford once wrote that sometime in the nineteenth century it became necessary to know how to read before one could truly see a building. Architecture had become referential, so a person needed a key in order to fully understand it. A Greek Revival house, for example, embodied a message about republican virtue that it helped to have at least some small knowledge of the classics to appreciate. To judge by the oceans of words that accompany prize-winning buildings today, the situation has evidently gotten much more complicated since Mumford's time. Nowadays you also have to be up on contemporary philosophy and literary theory in order to understand buildings. This seemed a great stroke of luck for me, since, as a former English major, I knew slightly more about these subjects than I did about building.

Take Peter Eisenman's Tokyo office tower. What had baffled me as a building, or model, began to make a certain amount of sense once I'd read the accompanying text. Eisenman's deconstructivist design is meant as "a kind of cultural critique of architectural stability and monumentality at a time when modern life itself is becoming increasingly contingent, tentative, and complex." Evidently the wrenching dislocations and foldings of space in this building will help office workers in Tokyo experience the dislocations and contingencies of contemporary life on a daily basis.*

About a lot of novel and even avant-garde architecture it's always been possible to say, Perhaps we just can't appreciate its beauty quite yet; maybe we'll have to catch up to it first. The label "Gothic," after all, was coined as a term of opprobrium for that style when it was new. It struck people as barbarous and ugly, so they named it for the detested Goths. But this new architecture is different. Making people uncomfortable is not merely the by-product of this style but its very purpose. It sets out to "deconstruct" the familiar categories we employ to organize our world: inside and outside, private and public, function and ornament, etc. Some of it does seem interesting as art, or maybe I should say, as text. But it seems to me it's one thing to disturb people in a museum or private home where anyone can choose not to venture, and quite another to set out to disorient office workers or conventioneers or passersby who have no choice in the matter. And who also haven't been given the chance to read the explanatory texts— the words upon words upon which so many of these structures have been built.

Likening this kind of architecture to a literary enterprise is not original with me. Eisenman himself claims that buildings are no more real than stories are, and in fact has urged his fellow architects to regard what they do as a form of "writing" rather than design. The old concept of design—as a process of creating forms that help negotiate between people and the real world—might

---

* Upsetting people in this manner is apparently taken as proof of success in this sort of architecture. According to a subsequent issue of *Progressive Architecture,* featuring a "post-occupancy critique" of a convention center Eisenman designed for the city of Cincinnati, the architect had been boasting that the "new spatial sensation" produced by his building had actually made one conventioneer throw up. (At the least, this represented a deconstruction of lunch.) But the boast turned out to be untrue, alas. After the reporter from *PA* tried in vain to track down the putative regurgitator, Eisenman was forced to concede he had been exaggerating.

have made sense when people still had some idea what "real" was, but now, "with reality in all its forms having been pre-empted by our mediated environment," architecture is free to reconceive itself as a literary art—personal, idiosyncratic, arbitrary.

For me, the irony of this situation was inescapable, a bad joke. I'd come to building looking for a way to get past words, only to learn from an influential contemporary architect that architecture was really just another form of writing. This was definitely a setback.

At first I assumed that this literary conception of architecture was a notion limited to deconstructivist architects and the editors of *Progressive Architecture*. But the more I read about contemporary architecture, the more widespread and uncritically accepted this idea seemed to be. Nobody seemed to have any trouble with the notion that language, of all things, is a suitable metaphor for architecture—that buildings "mean" in much the same way that words and sentences do, so that the proper way to experience a building is to "read" it. Postmodernism, the movement that preceded deconstruction in the parade of postwar architectural styles I found chronicled in the back issues of *PA*, promoted a completely different-looking kind of building, yet here too the underlying approach was essentially literary, and there was a lot of required reading. In this case, however, the syllabus was not deconstruction but semiotics—which happens to be the predecessor of deconstruction in the parade of postwar continental philosophies.

A quarter century before Peter Eisenman imported deconstruction to American architecture from Paris, Robert Venturi had imported semiotics, also from Paris. In *Learning from Las Vegas*, the immensely influential manifesto the Philadelphia architect and theorist published in 1972, he argued that architecture was not really so much about the articulation of space, as the modernists had believed, but about communication by means of signs, or symbols. Buildings constituted a form of media; they were cultural texts to be read. Venturi urged architects to recognize that what they were really doing was making "decorated sheds," and that it was the decorations, or symbols, that mattered most. The offspring of this theory was a slew of often very witty buildings self-consciously decorated with exaggerated (for ironic emphasis) columns, keystones, pediments, and, in Venturi's case especially, actual signs with words on them.

Working my way through recent architectural theory, I felt like I was back on familiar turf. In fact, Charlie's wordless little booklet about my hut was a lot more daunting than most of the buildings celebrated in the pages of *Progressive Architecture*, if only because the buildings in the magazine were based on texts with which I was at least glancingly familiar. But even if you didn't know the printed sources, with the help of the captions and manifestos you could read your way through them without too much trouble. They might be brick-and-mortar buildings, but they were also rivulets in the same information-age waters I'd always felt comfortable paddling around in.

And yet it hadn't been familiar waters I'd come to architecture looking for. I'd come because I wanted out of the tub. I'd come looking for something meatier than discourse, something nearer to the "views, sounds, and smells" of the material world that Hannah Arendt had celebrated. Buildings, I'd always assumed, had an especially strong claim on reality. Weren't they supposed to be one of those things in the world that gets pointed to, and not just another of the things that point? Yet it is precisely this quality that contemporary architecture seemed eager to deny.

I knew Charlie well enough to have a fair idea where he stood on these questions. He'd given me the subscription to *Progressive Architecture* as a way to define himself to me by counterexample: *This is everything I am not.* But he wasn't going to get into any arguments about it, because even to argue was to let himself be drawn onto the ground of words and theories, where he evidently had no wish to go. Of course this was *my* ground too, and Charlie's hesitance about me watching him work may have reflected a reasonable worry that I was going to somehow maneuver him out onto it. Only now did I understand that the exasperating wordlessness of his booklet, coming at the same time as the gift subscription to *PA*, had been meant as a gentle challenge. Charlie was asking me to choose, between the words and . . . what, exactly?

2. DRAWING

I drove up to Cambridge on a morning early in May to meet with Charlie about my building and, I hoped, to watch him begin to draw it. We met in his office, half a floor of a clapboard townhouse in Harvard Square, above a copy shop. His practice consisted of himself and a couple of freelance draftsmen, recent graduates of MIT's architecture school who came in, or not, depending on how much work was in-house. The undivided workspace was informal but orderly, a horseshoe of drafting tables set out beneath bookshelves stacked with cardboard models and large-format books. The designers I met looked like graduate students (blue jeans, sweaters, and sneakers), except for the stylish $300 eyeglasses.

At the time of my visit, the architecture profession was mired in a recession that had hit Boston-area architects particularly hard. The city's real estate market had collapsed, nobody was building, and with two local architecture schools continuing to graduate dozens of new architects each year, there simply were not enough commissions to go around. Charlie seemed to be getting by, however, with commissions for a couple of houses, a handful of residential renovation jobs, and the conversion of a building for an elementary school in Cambridge.

I had brought Charlie's book of images with me, and we started by working our way through it, sipping containers of coffee from the croissant shop downstairs. As Charlie talked over the pictures, often with a catching enthusiasm, they immediately became less opaque. For one thing, I realized I had overcomplicated their import. I'd be puzzling over what a sprawling New England farmhouse could possibly have to do with my little shack when all he had wanted me to notice was the vine-tangled trellis over the porch, which he thought we might want to try on the window facing the ornery neighbor.

"That's a great solution for a place where you want light but the view really stinks. The vines filter the sunlight nicely, too, since the leaves are always moving." Charlie could be fervent talking about a window, describing the tone of the light it admitted to a room, or how flinging it open was apt to make you feel about life. He seemed so much more articulate in person than on the phone, and as I watched him talk about these images, hands and brows and even shoulders in almost constant motion, I realized that Charlie's is a kind of full-body eloquence.

Only a few of the images were meant to be taken as literally as the vine-covered window. The reason he'd included the European townhouse that resembled a cat, for example, was because he felt my building should have an anthropomorphic façade. "It makes sense for our guy to have a strong face, since this is going to be a one-man house." Okay, but a cat? "Hey. Don't be so literal," Charlie grinned. "This is just a reminder to me, something to think about when I'm drawing the elevation." He explained that many of the images in the book had a similar purpose: They were cues to help him focus on issues he might otherwise lose track of in the design process—ways of thinking about windows, doors, ceilings, and roofs, the various ways a building can meet the ground.

"Like this door here—" He pointed to a picture of a formal Edwardian townhouse entrance. "Now this is obviously completely wrong for our building, but it's such a fantastic example of *doorness.* It's a reminder I need to deal with the whole issue of just what kind of experience the entrance to our building is going to be—

should it be a public or a private kind of thing? Do we want to be inviting people up here with some kind of ceremonial front door like this one here, or do we want to maybe put them off a bit with something more backdoorish?" We talked about that for a while, and agreed the door should definitely be around back, where you wouldn't see it until you'd stepped around the big rock. Then Charlie suggested we try to place the door on one of the thick walls: "That way, the entrance to the building becomes a real passage. As you walk in you'll feel the great mass of that wall of books surrounding you." He hunched his shoulders close, as if he were squeezing through the stacks in a library.

Paging through the book with Charlie, I began to see that the real subject of these pictures was not architectural ideas or styles so much as architectural *experiences*. Each picture evoked what a particular kind of place or space felt like, they were poetic that way, and it was the sensual nature of each experience, more than any purely visual or aesthetic details, that Charlie meant to call my attention to.

Turning to the picture of the Caribbean porch with the thatched roof and nonexistent walls, he talked about the sharp juxtaposition of the low, sheltering roof line and the wide open spaces underneath it. "Isn't this fantastic? It reminds me of putting the top down on a convertible, that explosion of light and space you get the moment the roof flies up, only here it's the walls that vanish. Makes me think of Frank Lloyd Wright, too, the way his strong roofs meet those light, dematerialized walls so that the space seems to race outward, right through them. We could do something like that." I realized that the reason vernacular shacks and barns could cohabit so happily in Charlie's booklet with examples of sophisticated architecture is that, for him, when they work, both draw on the same elemental feelings about space.

I asked Charlie about this. "People do seem to have some very basic responses to places and kinds of spaces," he said, picking his words with care as he stepped gingerly out onto the ice of architectural theory. "I do happen to believe that there's a basic vocabulary of 'buildingness' that we all share. This is what I try to work with—they're my tubes of paint. And that's really all this little booklet is about: singling out a handful of strong spatial experiences that might belong in your building." Charlie used the word "vocabulary" to describe these architectural elements, but it seemed to me they could scarcely be less literary. He wasn't talking about our interpretation of architectural conventions so much as our unconscious experiences of space—the sort of immediate, poetic responses to place that Bachelard chronicled in *The Poetics of Space,* a book that turned out to be close to Charlie's heart.

I asked him if anyone else had written about this face of architecture, which seemed such a long way from the world I'd been reading about in *PA.* He mentioned Christopher Alexander, a somewhat unorthodox Bay Area architect who has tried systematically to analyze and catalog all the forms in architecture's vocabulary, almost as if they were parts of nature and he were an obsessed naturalist.

Alexander calls these forms "patterns," and his best-known book, *A Pattern Language**, published in 1977, is essentially a compilation of 253 of them in a phone-book-thick volume that reads like a vast field guide or encyclopedia. Each pattern is numbered and named ("159: Light on Two Sides of Every Room"), de-

---

* It's curious that both Charlie and Alexander would use a linguistic metaphor to describe architecture's fundamental elements. Alexander's conception of architecture is no more literary than Charlie's—his patterns are clearly not signs or metaphors. Perceiving a pattern is less a matter of interpretation than experience; indeed, many of his patterns (like "Watching the World Go By") are activities as much as material forms. My hunch is that Charlie and Alexander are both thinking of language in only the most rudimentary and old-fashioned sense, as a system that makes it possible to combine a finite number of basic building blocks into an infinite number of more complicated structures. In Alexander's conception, words are not nearly as ambiguous or arbitrary as modern philosophy has taught us to regard them.

fined in a sentence ("People will always gravitate to those rooms which have light on two sides, and leave the rooms which are lit from one side unused and empty"), and illustrated with a photograph or drawing. Charlie hadn't exactly read *A Pattern Language*, he admitted, but he'd browsed around in it enough to decide that the definitions and illustrations were apt and even useful, and he suggested I have a look.

My first impression of *A Pattern Language* was that it reminded me of Charlie's booklet a bit, except that there were long, interesting captions to accompany the photographs, as well as an overarching theory. Like the pictures in Charlie's book, Alexander's were strongly evocative of the experience of place: One showed a casement window flung open to embrace an early-morning street scene that reminded me of Paris readying to greet the workday; another, a trellis of bean vines that filigreed the sunlight coming through the window of a shack. There were big pine-plank tables in farmhouse kitchens you wanted to pull a chair up to, and front porches that seemed to say, here's a sweet place to watch the world go by.

The images were well chosen and immediately appealing, yet the text made clear that there was something more here than a collection of nice places. We were told, in fact, that the "patterns" depicted in these images revealed profound truths about the world and human nature. Indeed, Alexander states that the discovery of any one of these patterns—of something like "light on two sides of every room" or "entrance transition"—is "as hard as anything in theoretical physics." In a strange and wonderful way, *A Pattern Language* manages to combine a rich poetry of everyday life with the monomania of someone who believes he has found a key to the universe. I suspect Charlie had soaked up the former and skipped over the latter.

With my own well-established weakness for theories, I wasn't about to do anything of the kind. I dug in. Alexander contends (in both *A Pattern Language* and a more theoretical companion volume called *The Timeless Way of Building*) that the most successful built forms share certain essential attributes with forms in nature—with things like trees and waves and animals. Both natural and man-made forms serve to reconcile conflicting forces (a tree's need to stand up with the fact of gravity, say, or a person's conflicting urges for privacy and social contact); the forms that do this best are the ones that endure. You might say that Alexander is an architectural Charles Darwin, since he believes that good form represents a successful adaptation to a given environment.

Consider the living room of a house, Alexander writes. Here the conflicting forces are not physical but psychological: the desire of family members for a sense of belonging and the simultaneous need of individuals for a measure of privacy and time apart. The pattern that will resolve this basic conflict (which Alexander says lies at the heart not only of family life but of social life in general) he calls "Alcoves": "To give a group a chance to be together, as a group, a room must also give them the chance to be alone, in one's and two's in the same space." This is accomplished by creating "small places at the edge of any common room. . . . These alcoves should be large enough for two people to sit, chat, or play, and sometimes large enough to contain a desk or a table." The pattern of an alcove off of a communal space (which also shows up in libraries, restaurants, and public squares) is as natural and right and self-sustaining as the pattern of ripples in a patch of windblown sand.

It follows that architectural beauty is not a subjective or a trivial matter for Alexander. "Everybody loves window seats, bay windows, and big windows with low sills and comfortable chairs drawn up to them," he declares in the pattern "Window Place," which follows "Alcoves" in *A Pattern Language*. A room lacking this pattern—even if it has a window and comfortable chair somewhere in it—will "keep you in a state of perpetual unresolved conflict and tension." That's because when you enter the room you will feel torn between the desire to sit down and be comfortable and the desire to move toward the light. Only a window place that combines the comfortable spot to sit with the source of sunlight can resolve this tension. For Alexander, our sense that rooms containing such places are beautiful is much more than "an aesthetic whim"; rather, a window place, like an alcove off a common room, represents an objectively successful adaptation to a given social and physical context.

Whether or not you are willing to travel quite this far with Alexander, his book fairly brims with patterns that seem sensible and ring with a certain poetic or psychological truth. I'd never thought about it before, but having windows on two sides of a room *does* seem to make the difference between a lifeless and an appealing room. The reason this is so, Alexander hypothesizes, is that a dual light source allows us to see things more intricately, especially the finer details of facial expression and gesture. Similarly, there is something vital about the experience of arrival captured in the pattern "Entrance Transition," which calls for a transitional space at the entrance to a building—a covered porch, or a curving path brushing by a lilac, or some other slight change of view or texture underfoot before one reaches the door. Alexander suggests that people need this sort of transitional space and time in order to shed their "street behaviors" and settle "into the more intimate spirit appropriate to a house." Sometimes Alexander sounds less like an architect than a novelist. I say that not only because he is a good student of human nature, but because he brings a sense of narrative—of time—to the design of space.

I realized that Charlie and I were sensing the need for just such an "entrance transition" when we decided to locate the door in back. Stepping around the big rock and turning into the site would create the very interlude Alexander is talking about, offering a change in perspective and a moment to prepare before coming inside. It was startling to see just how many of the things I asked for in my letter, and how many of the images in Charlie's book, show up in *A Pattern Language.* "Thick walls," for example, turns out to be an important pattern: "Most of the identity of a dwelling lies in or near its surfaces—in the 3 or 4 feet near the walls." These should be thick enough to accommodate shelves, cabinets, displays, lamps, built-in furniture—all those nooks and niches that allow people to leave their mark on a place. "Each house will have a memory," Alexander writes, and the personalities of its inhabitants are "written in the thickness of the walls." So maybe I hadn't been that far off, imagining the walls of my hut as an auxiliary brain.

≡

After we had spent a couple of hours going through the book of images, using them to narrow my choices and refine our idea of the building, Charlie took out a roll of parchment-colored tracing paper, drew a length of it across his drafting table, and began to draw. He worked in ink to start, sketching rapidly in rough, scribbly lines, discarding a drawing and tearing off a new length of paper any time he didn't like what he was seeing. If there was anything in a sketch worth saving, he'd start the new drawing by loosely tracing over that part of the rejected one; in this way a process of trial and error unfolded swiftly and smoothly, the good ideas getting carried forward from one generation of drawing to the next, the bad ones falling by the wayside.

At first, Charlie worked exclusively in plan, ignoring for the time being what the building might look like from the outside. He started with my desk, which we'd decided should carry all the way across the front of the building, where it could overlook the pond and the house. To determine its dimensions, Charlie inventoried the things I liked to keep on my desk and then asked me to extend my arms out to the sides. To that wingspan (six feet) he added the depth of a bookshelf on each end (two feet): this gave us the width of the building. Charlie now turned to the Golden Section to obtain its length, multiplying eight feet by the factor 1.618, which comes to 12.9. He sketched a rectangle eight feet by thirteen, roughed in the big rock to its right, and declared, "There it is: your ur-house."

We had talked about the Golden Section earlier, when we'd come to that section in the book of images. Charlie told me he often resorted to the ratio when he had to make a decision about the proportions of a space. He'd devoted a couple of pages to it in the booklet because he thought the Golden Section seemed particularly fitting for this building, since it was to house someone who liked to write about nature. When I offered a puzzled look, he explained that, among other things, the Golden Section is a bridge joining the worlds of architecture and nature. "The same proportioning system that works in buildings also shows up in trees, leaves, in the spirals of seashells and sunflowers, and in the human body." He hoisted his eyebrows, lowered his voice: "It's everywhere."

But wasn't this an awfully mystical way to determine the proportions of my building?

"Hey. It works. More often than not, rooms with Golden Section proportions feel right." Charlie stressed that he's not a slave to the system; should he find he needs a couple more feet in the length of the building, for example, he'll dispense with it. "But all other things being equal, I'll use it, because I'm convinced there's something there."

I was surprised that such an occult proportioning system hadn't gone out with the Enlightenment, or modernism, but Charlie rattled off a long list of modern architects who'd sworn by it, including two as different as Le Corbusier and Frank Lloyd Wright. Even to contemporary designers not at all given to mysticism or numerology, the Golden Section seems to retain some value as a pattern, or type—something to fall back on when faced with a decision about proportions, providing a bit of shelter, perhaps, from what Kevin Lynch, the writer and city planner, once called "the anxieties of the open search."

For the next hour, Charlie worked variations on this basic rectangle, now moving the daybed from the east wall to a bay on the south wall, now switching places between the daybed and the stove. At one point he experimented with the idea of turning the front of the building into a screened-in porch, while moving the desk to the north wall. But that meant it would look right out on the giant boulder, and when I mentioned that this seemed like a good recipe for writer's block, he quickly dropped that idea.

Sheet after sheet, Charlie moved around the elements we'd settled on—desk, daybed, porch, stove, bookshelves, chair—like pieces on a chessboard, talking the whole time as if we were inside the game and the pieces were animate. "This guy here," he'd say, pointing to the chair, "really wants to be over there by the stove, but if we move him, like so, then the daybed can't go on the same wall because code says you need at least three feet of clearance to a combustible on either side of your stove." He started to draw it anyway. "Unless, that is, you decide not to bother with a building permit—" he looked at me hopefully; this wouldn't be the last time Charlie tried to keep on going after one of his ideas ran up against some practical consideration. I told him to stick to code. "Okay, okay, so . . ."—he tears off another length of tracing paper—"let's move the bay window for the daybed to the south wall, where it's really going to want that shady trellis"—he scribbled a dense tangle of lines over the window—"and then put the door on the east end, the stove back over here . . . This just might work."

As he tested each new arrangement of elements in plan, Charlie would narrate a procession through the imaginary space taking shape at the end of his felt-tip. "Now I approach the building this way, turning right up here past the rock, which is hiding the big view from me, that's perfect, and then I step into the building, passing through our thick wall here . . . Good." Thinking, narrating, and drawing seemed to proceed almost in lockstep, the process now pushing, now following, the prow of black ink over the sheet of paper. His line danced across the page with a quality that managed to look both sure-footed and provisional at the same time, doubling back on itself to correct an angle or try out a new dimension, then flying off to scribble a shelf full of books while its author contemplated his next move. Swift, buoyant, heedless for now about being neat or right, it was a line that seemed to say, "Okay, so how about *this*?" Charlie's words hustled to keep pace with its improvisations.

"So now I've arrived," he continued, his pen swinging a door open to the left. "And right there in front of me is the daybed with the bay window behind it, looking out through our clematis vine, all that filtered south light. Good, good, good. Then I turn to my right, and boom, there's the big view down to the pond—that's very strong, the surprise as I turn into that view. So let's make the most of it, carry that window wall to wall like this, run it the entire length of the desk. Nice. Uh-oh"—he flashes a panicked look, eyebrows rocketing—"I don't see the porch! Where am I going to put *that* guy? And it looks like that stove and chair are going to be in my way as I move toward the desk. It's starting to get a little crowded in here." He tore off another length of tracing paper.

Now Charlie seemed stuck, and while he sat there rubbing his chin, a half-dozen rejected schemes spread out in front of him, I opened the booklet to the photograph of the miniature bungalow with the glassed-in room squatting over its front porch. Maybe we could go up, like this, I suggested. Charlie told me a little about the house in the picture, evidently a favorite. It was in a campground on Cape Cod called Nonquit, a summer community his grandparents had been members of, where Charlie had spent time as a child. He spoke affectionately of the place, and especially of the strong, eccentric architecture there, which he still sometimes returned to admire and, occasionally, borrow from. Every house was different, Charlie said, idiosyncratic but without straining to be. They'd been built at the turn of the century by Beaux Arts–trained architects working in vernacular American idioms—stick, shingle style, bungalow. What he admired most about these buildings was their simultaneous inventiveness and unpretentiousness, qualities not easily combined.

"The houses have a certain propriety I've always associated with my grandparents." These were the Quakers on his mother's side. "They're very sophisticated buildings—a dozen different ideas in each—yet they'd much rather be thought of as plain than risk seeming the least bit affected. But there are layers upon layers here if you look. You're welcome to uncover as much, or as little, as you want." Charlie seemed to prize this notion of propriety in people and buildings equally.

Now he seized on the idea of a small second story, and set off in a whole new direction, drawing a square, about five foot on a side, in the middle of our rectangle—a tower, essentially, that would rise above the main room and accommodate either the daybed or the desk. I told Charlie about my tree house, which the tower he was drawing reminded me of. We were suddenly on much trickier ground, having now to factor in a half-dozen new and relatively inflexible elements, like the clearance beneath the second story ("How tall are you? Let's see if we can get away with seven feet under here") and some means of access to it that wouldn't eat up too much space downstairs. A staircase would take up nearly as much square footage as we were adding, so we played with the idea of using a library ladder on a track, which would slide right into the thick wall and out of the way.

The rest of the morning was taken up elaborating the tower scheme. After we had settled on what seemed to be a workable arrangement in plan—my desk lining the glazed walls of the tower, the front of the house below becoming a porch, with the stove and sitting area directly beneath the tower, and the daybed still occupying a bay window curving out from the south wall downstairs—Charlie declared that the moment of truth had arrived. It was time to see what this thing was going to look like in elevation.

Still working in ink, Charlie sketched what looked like a miniature bungalow with a boxy tower rising up through the middle of its roof to form a second, parallel gable above it, like so:

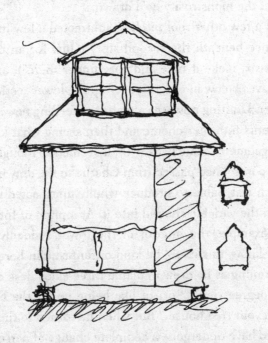

"Well, he's definitely his own guy," Charlie said, drumming his Uniball fine-point on the edge of his drafting table as he appraised the elevation. It did seem vaguely anthropomorphic, with the makings of a strong face. But I wondered if maybe it wasn't too public a face—the kind you'd expect to meet in a village, or in a campground like Nonquit, but perhaps not alone in the woods.

Charlie said it was too soon to tell. "At a certain point, you have to start getting real about a scheme—start drawing it in elevation with actual dimensions and roof pitches. That's when an idea that might seem to work in a rough drawing can take on a whole new

personality—or fall apart." Now Charlie switched to pencil, drawing to scale a very precise set of parallel roof lines, one directly
above the other. First he tried the same fairly shallow thirty-degree
roof pitch our house had, thinking that this might set up a dialogue
between the two buildings. But it soon became clear that this pitch
would not give me enough headroom upstairs without making the
tower so tall as to overwhelm the rest of the building. Charlie
chuckled at the monstrosity he'd drawn.

He tried a few other roof pitches, subtracted a few inches from
the clearance beneath the second story ("Just for an experiment
let's try six-six, make it nice and cozy under there"), and length-
ened the eaves below in order to beef up the lower section relative
to the tower. Drafting now was a matter of feeding new angles and
measurements into the scheme and then seeing what kind of elevation the geometry came back with; it seemed as though a certain
amount of control had passed from Charlie to the drawing process
itself, which was liable to produce wholly unexpected results depending on the variables he fed into it. At a pitch of forty-five degrees, for example, the interior of the tower suddenly began to
work. "You know, this could be kind of fantastic in here," Charlie
said, brightening as he drew in plan a three-sided desk command-
ing a 270-degree view. "Sort of like being up on the bridge of a
ship—or in your tree house." But when he turned to the elevation
it seemed to have undergone a complete change of personality. No
longer a funky campground bungalow, the building had gone back
in time half a century and acquired a somewhat Gothic-Victorian
aspect, with its steeply pitched roof and slender, upward-thrusting
tower. A woodland setting now seemed to suit this house, it was
true, but unfortunately it was the woods of the Brothers Grimm:
The elevation now suggested a gingerbread cottage. It had gotten
cute. Charlie scowled at the drawing. "It's a hobbit house!"

But the tower scheme had its own momentum now, so Charlie
kept at it, playing with the elevation while trying to keep the plan
more or less intact, deploying a whole bag of tricks to rid the build-

ing of its fairy-tale associations and balance the relative weight of top and bottom. He abbreviated the eaves, beefed up the timbers below while lightening them above, overthrew the symmetry of the façade, and drew in a series of unexpectedly big windows, all of which served to undercut the house's "hobbitiness." By the time we decided to break for lunch, the elevation had lost any trace of cuteness, which Charlie clearly felt was the peril in designing such a miniature building. "This is starting to look like something," Charlie declared at last, by which of course he meant exactly the opposite: The building no longer looked like anything you could readily give a name to—neither bungalow nor gingerbread cottage. The building was once again its own guy. Whether it was *my* guy neither of us felt quite sure. So we decided to put the drawing away for a while, see how it looked to us in a few days.

By now, Charlie and I had traveled pretty far down this particular road, having invested so much work in the tower scheme. But as I drove home to Connecticut later that afternoon, I began to have doubts about it. Mainly I wondered if the building wasn't getting too big and complicated. My shack in the woods had turned into a two-story house, and I wasn't sure if it was something I could afford, much less build myself; it certainly didn't look inexpensive or idiot-proof. When I got home that evening, I walked out to the site, and recalled Charlie's remark about propriety as I tried to imagine the building in place. Out here on this wooded, rocky hillside, in the middle of this fallen-down farm, it seemed clear that the building he'd drawn would call too much attention to itself. In this particular context, it lacked propriety. Charlie had devised a scheme that would give me everything I'd asked for, it was true, but perhaps that was the problem. Somehow, the building seemed to be getting away from us.

≡

Charlie phoned me first. "I'm starting all over," he announced, much to my relief. "There's no reason we can't get the things you want here—a couple of distinct spaces, a desk, a daybed, a stove, and some kind of porch—without going to two stories." Drawing the tower scheme had been a valuable exercise, Charlie said. It had helped him to think through all the programmatic elements by getting them down on paper. But now he wanted to go back to the basic eight-by-thirteen rectangle, see if he couldn't figure out some way to condense all the elements and patterns I wanted into that frame.

"We need to tame this thing—impose some tighter rules. That usually produces better architecture anyway. I can't lose sight of the basic simplicity of our program here: it's a hut in the woods, a place for you to work. It is not a second house."

He started talking about a four-by-eight-foot playhouse he was building for his boys in Tamworth, New Hampshire, where he spent weekends in a converted chicken coop that had been in his family for three generations. The playhouse, which was in the woods up behind the house, consisted of four gigantic timber corner posts set on boulders and crowned with a gable roof framed out of undressed birch logs.

"We could do something like that here: a primitive hut, basically, with a post-and-beam frame. That way, the walls don't bear any load, which gives us a lot of freedom. We could do some walls thick, others thin. I could even work out some sort of removable wall system, or perhaps windows that disappear into the walls, or up into the ceiling, so that in the summer the whole building turns into a porch."

Charlie seemed full of ideas now, some of them—like the disappearing windows—sounding fairly complex, and others so primitive as to be worrisome. For example, he wasn't sure that my building needed a foundation. We could just sink pressure-treated corner posts into the ground, or maybe seat the whole building on four boulders, like his boys' playhouse. Wouldn't the frost heave the boulders every winter? That's no big deal, he said; you rent a house jack and jack the building up in the spring. Charlie was bringing a very different approach to the project now, trying radically to simplify it, to get it back to first principles after the complications of the tower scheme. Which was fine with me, though I told him that I definitely did not want a building that had to be jacked up every April.

From our conversations, I knew that the primitive hut was a powerful image for Charlie, as indeed it has been for many architects at least since the time of Vitruvius. Almost all of the classic architecture treatises I'd read—by Vitruvius, Alberti, Laugier and, more recently, Le Corbusier and Wright—start out with a vivid account of the building of the First Shelter, which serves these author-architects as a myth of architecture's origins in the state of nature; it also provides a theoretical link between the work of building and the art of architecture. Depending on the author, the primal shelter might be a tent or cave or a wooden post-and-beam hut with a gable roof. More often than not, the architect proceeds to draw a direct line of historical descent from his version of the primitive hut to the style of architecture he happens to practice, thereby implying that this kind of building alone carries nature's seal of approval. If an architect favors neoclassical architecture over Gothic, for example, chances are his primitive hut will bear a close resemblance to a Greek temple built out of tree trunks.

Literature has its primitive huts too—think of Robinson Crusoe's or Thoreau's: simple dwellings for not-so-simple characters who find in such a building a good vantage point from which to cast a gimlet eye upon society. The sophisticate's primitive hut becomes a tool with which to explore civilized man's relation to nature and criticize whatever in the contemporary scene strikes the author as artificial or decadent. The idea, in literature and architecture alike, seems to be that a decadent society or style of building can be renewed and refreshed by closer contact with nature, by a return to the first principles and truthfulness embodied in the primitive hut.

For Charlie, the appeal of the hut seemed a good deal less ideological than all that. To him, the image bespoke plain, honest structure; an architecture made out of the materials at hand; a simple habitation carved out of the wilderness; and an untroubled relationship to nature. He had told me about reading the eighteenth-century *philosophe* Marc-Antoine Laugier's *Essay on Architecture* in architecture school and coming across the etching of a primitive hut on its frontispiece: Charles Eisen's "Allegory of Architecture Returning to its Natural Model," which depicts four trees in a rectangle, their branches knitted together to form a leafy, sheltering gable above. "It's a completely romantic idea," Charlie said. "But it's kind of wonderful, too, the image of these four trees giving themselves up to us as the four corners of a shelter—this dream of a perfect marriage between man and nature."

A few weeks later, I received a somewhat cryptic fax from Charlie:

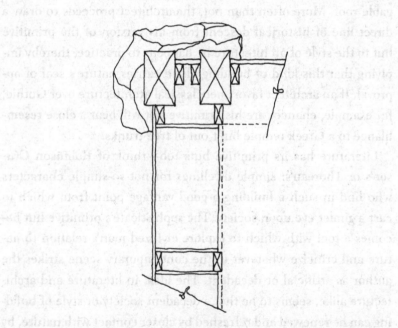

When I reached him late that afternoon, he sounded excited. "So what do you think?" I confessed I didn't really understand the drawing.

"Oh. Well, what you've got there is the detail for the southwest corner of your building. I've been working on it for a week, and this morning it finally came together."

The corner detail?

"No, the whole scheme."

I asked when I could see the rest of it.

"This detail's all I've drawn so far. But that's our *parti*, right there—the solution to the problem, in a nutshell. The rest should be fairly easy."

I still didn't get it.

"See, the problem I've been having with this hut all along is with the thickness of the corner posts." Charlie was deep inside the new scheme now, and his explanation came in a rush. "Basically, the idea is to do thick walls on the long sides, thin ones front and back. What this does is give the building a strong directionality—it becomes almost a kind of chute, funneling all that space coming down through our site toward the pond."

He proceeded to explain how the thickness of the posts set up the thickness of our interior walls, which meant the posts would have to be a foot square at a minimum if the walls were going to work as bookshelves. But in fact they had to be a couple of inches thicker than that, since he wanted them to "come proud" of the walls—stand out from the building's skin, in order to retain their "postness."

"So already we're up to fifteen, sixteen inches square, which is one fat post. I tried drawing it—*way* too chunky. You'd need a crane to haul it out there.

"But what if instead I go to a *pair* of posts, six by six, say, with three or four inches of wall between them? That gives me my fifteen inches easily, but without any of that chunkiness." A single fat corner post would also have suggested that all four of our walls were equally thick, he explained, while a pair of posts at each corner in front would imply that only the long walls directly behind them are thick; by comparison the short walls between the double posts at either end will seem thin, an impression he planned to underscore by filling them with glass.

"There was one more piece of the puzzle, though, which didn't hit me till this morning. Instead of two square posts, what if I go to six-by-tens and run them lengthwise? This way our corner could articulate the directionality of the building at the same time it sets up the whole idea of thick versus thin walls—enclosure one way, openness the other. That's what I mean about the whole *parti* being right here in a nutshell."

Charlie might have been able to tease an entire building out of his corner detail, but I couldn't see it, not yet. I might as well have been trying to picture a face by looking at a handful of genes in a microscope. I did notice, however, that Charlie's corner post sat on a rock, and I asked him about that; I wasn't going to need a house jack, was I? He assured me there was a conventional footing underneath the rock. The rock was his way of hiding the ungainly concrete pier we'd need to support the double posts. Stone footings also seemed right for the site. "What else could a big wooden post standing next to a boulder wear on its feet?"

Charlie said he still had a few big issues to resolve, and the elevations to draw. "It's a tight fit in there, and I haven't figured out how I'm going to resolve the tops of the double posts, or how I'm going to make our thin walls disappear. But the hard part's done. I should have something for you to look at in a week."

3. THE DESIGN

Charlie drove down to present his design over the Fourth of July weekend. Sunday morning, out on the porch, he unfurled a single large blueprint that he had prepared with the help of Don Knerr, a young associate in his office. The drawing showed the big rock with the floor plan of the hut next to it and, orbiting around that, the four elevations and two cross-section views. They'd also sketched in some trees for atmosphere, and a curl of smoke rising from the stovepipe. I noticed the building was called a "Writing House" on the blueprint, an accurate enough but somewhat grand-sounding name it would take me awhile to make my own.

My first impression was of how simple this building looked, considering all the thought and work that had gone into it. Here in plan was a basic rectangular box, and in elevation a square crowned by an isosceles right triangle: a house as a child might have drawn it. But as Charlie began to walk me through the drawings, narrating a trip through spaces that seemed as vivid to him as the porch we were sitting on, the simple hut began to disclose a few of its layers of complexity. Others I wouldn't encounter for several months yet, not until I'd begun to build it.

"The building is basically a pair of bookshelves holding up a roof," Charlie began, a catch of nervousness in his voice. "It's about living between two substantial walls that hold everything you're about—or at least, everything this building's about—and which channel all the air and space and energy streaming through this site." As Charlie had predicted it would, the facts of the site had determined key elements of the building's design. Its directionality, for example, was "given to us" by the flow of space between the rock and the hedgerow. The rock itself had dictated a building of great strength, Charlie explained; a lightly framed shack or gazebo would have been overwhelmed by the boulder, which "wanted a very beefy, post-and-beamy companion." Yet there were also a couple of elements in the design that promised to feel extremely light and open to nature. The roof was a membrane of cedar shingles thin and delicate enough to transmit the tap of rain, Charlie said, and the two end walls would virtually disappear when I opened the main windows.

In plan, Charlie had indeed teased an entire building out of his original corner detail. Between the pairs of six-by-ten posts at either end of the rectangle ran foot-thick walls the length of the building; these were the bookshelves that held up the roof. Each of the short sides of the rectangle, the front and back, was dominated by a big, horizontal awning window that carried from post to post. These windows were hinged at the top to open inward; raised overhead and then hooked to a chain hanging down from the ridge beam, they would disappear into the ceiling, almost like garage doors. Across the front, or west wall of the building was the main part of the desk; directly opposite it, on the east wall, was the daybed, which hadn't ended up on the thick wall after all. That's because those walls had been interrupted by a pair of steps, which divided a lower work area in front from a smaller raised landing in back that accommodated the daybed and the entrance. In plan the steps divided the room into a square (the landing) and a rectangle that appeared to have Golden Section proportions; they also served to rhyme the floor of the building with the slope of the site.

Judith joined us at the table, carefully settling her eighth-month frame into the chair across from Charlie; Isaac would be born a few weeks later. "So this is where my child is going to go to smoke pot in fifteen years," she said, patting her belly. "No," Charlie smiled, pointing to the daybed on the blueprint. "This is where he loses his virginity." Neither prospect had ever occurred to me, but of course my building would outlive my intentions for it in all sorts of unforeseeable ways. It was going to be a thing in the world, not just an idea in my or Charlie's head.

Charlie walked us through the design. After stepping around the big rock, you would enter the building through a low door on the thick wall, arriving on the upper landing. To the left was the daybed, which would have a dropped ceiling above it finished in narrow strips of clear pine; the idea was to make this space somewhat more refined and intimate than the rest of the building, Charlie explained, a room within a room. Directly ahead as you entered would be a double casement window cut into the thick wall and obscured by a trellis smothered in vines.

From the little landing, the space stepped down into the work area, following the grade of the ground below. Charlie pointed out that since the height of the ceiling stayed constant, as you come down the steps "you're going to feel the space lift from your shoulders"—a slight shift in mood. The workspace was dominated by a deep L-shaped desk that ran across the entire front and along most of the north wall, where there would be a little casement window tucked right into the bookshelf at desk height and opening directly on the rock. This window would allow me to see anybody approaching without getting up from my desk. Charlie said he'd placed the big window down low over the desk so that the pond wouldn't come completely into view until you stepped down into the work area. "And then, when you pop those two awning windows open, the front and back walls are basically going to vanish, leaving nothing but air post to post. It's the top-down-on-the-convertible effect we talked about, the whole building transformed into a screened-in porch."

The thick walls would feel as strongly present as the thin ones would seem ephemeral, Charlie said. These were divided into five bays approximately thirty inches wide; three in the lower space, two above. Each bay was defined by what Charlie called a "fin wall," a twelve-inch-deep section of plywood-faced wall jutting in perpendicularly from the building's plywood sheathing. These dividers would run floor to ceiling, giving the walls their thickness and anchoring the bookshelves. Along with the rafters, the fin walls composed the building's skeleton, which was entirely exposed. At the top of the wall each fin met a four-by-six rafter that carried the frame up to the spine and then continued down the other side, where it met another fin wall, almost as though the whole space were suspended within a wooden rib cage.

In the cross-section drawings, you could see how the thick walls did most of the work of the building. Many of the bays were filled with bookshelves, but others held such things as the stove, a stack of logs, the desk, two of the windows, the door, a nook for my computer, and another for stationery and supplies. It looked like I could reach just about all these spaces from my desk chair—retrieve a book, feed the stove, crack a window. Charlie had given me the cockpit I'd asked for. The building was indeed boatlike, not only in its radical economy of space, but also in its ribbed frame and pronounced directionality.

The front of the building looked fairly straightforward in elevation, though it too held layers it would take me awhile to appreciate. Two pairs of thick Douglas fir posts rose from rock bases on either side of a broad window that was divided into six square panes, three over three. The window was capped by a wooden visor, and above that a gable, which was pierced by a pair of tiny windows directly beneath the peak. These matched the windows under the peak of the main house, striking a slight family resemblance between the two buildings. To my eye the elevation made no obvious stylistic or historical reference, though with its clean geometry and strong frontality you would have to say it leaned closer to the classical than the Gothic. The front elevation gave an impression of being open (even without a front door), resolute, frank, and somewhat masculine—a fit companion for the boulder it would sit next to.

Charlie said that drawing the elevation had been a struggle, that the double posts had given him a lot of trouble. A single post would have been easy to resolve, Charlie explained; simply run it up into the frame of the building, so that it turns into the gable's first rafter. But how do you terminate an inside post? If it travels up into the gable, it looks like a mistake, "or some kind of Gothic stick-style reference." The obvious solution would have been to cap the posts with some kind of capital, or a cornice running across the front of the building. "But that immediately says 'Greek Revival'— makes the building seem like some postmodern temple plopped out here in the woods. I wanted to avoid those kinds of associations at all costs."

I asked him why that was so important.

"Because I wanted this building to be it's own person. If I'd used the Greek Revival solution, it would have been too literal, too referential. The building immediately becomes part of a specific discourse. You'd look at it and start thinking about Venturi, about postmodernism and irony. It's also just too easy. Suddenly you no longer even have to *look* at the building—one glance at the Greek Revival sign on the front and you've got it, you're done. That's much too fast, too cerebral. I want you to experience this thing, not read it."

It was the wooden visor that had given Charlie a way to resolve his corner detail without falling into postmodern mannerism. "This little guy here does a lot for us," he explained. As a practical matter, it meant I could leave the window open in the rain, and in the late afternoon it would keep the sun out of my eyes. In formal terms, it actually *is* a kind of cornice, since it runs across the base of the pediment and caps the double columns. But a visor is so emphatically casual that it immediately shrugs off any classical associations, defusing any hint of formality or pretension in the elevation. "If this thing's a temple," Charlie said, "it's a temple that wears a baseball cap."

I recalled the notion of architectural propriety we'd discussed in Boston. Charlie had taken pains to make certain that the building not come off the least bit flashy, though often he seemed to have arrived at his simple effects by a very complicated route. My building may have been a primitive hut—a wooden rectangle of space defined by four corner posts and a gable roof—but it was a most sophisticated primitive hut, a considered object from the ground (where its "simple" rock footings disguised modern concrete piers) up to its peak, where the two inconspicuous windows peered out at the world, knowingly.

"I took what you said to heart," Charlie said at one point near the end of his presentation. "That your building should seem fairly straightforward outside, yet have a kind of density within. We certainly could have done something a lot zippier in elevation—the tower scheme, say. Or we could have put a metal roof on it instead of these cedar shingles. But how self-conscious do we want to say we are?" This seemed like a particularly telling way for Charlie to phrase his sense of propriety. It suggested that self-consciousness, and complexity and sophistication, are given, inescapable—this was, after all, a building designed in the last decade of the twentieth century, a "primitive hut" in the woods that will nevertheless house a computer and a modem and a fax machine, not to mention my own word-bound, hypertheoretical self.

=

With only a few small modifications, this was the building I would set out to build a few months later. Charlie had managed to give me everything I had asked for without compromising the basic idea of a hut, and he had done so with an impressive economy, even a measure of poetry, and by using the most basic of materials: a frame of Douglas fir, plywood walls, a skin of cedar shingles. The building also promised, at least on paper, to suit its site as well as it suited me, to make a fit companion for that boulder. It appeared that Charlie had found a way to harmonize my wishes with the facts of this particular landscape.

That evening, after Charlie had left for Boston, I reread the first letter I'd sent him, setting forth my many tangled wishes for the building. The desk, daybed, bookshelves, stove, sitting area, even the porch (or at least, a sense of "porchness")—all the elements and patterns I'd specified were there. But instead of simply adding them up or stringing them together, Charlie had, like a boat builder, found intelligent ways to layer a great many different things into the confines of a single eight-by-thirteen-foot room. One pattern overlapped another, so that the thick walls were enlisted to help create the sense of an entrance transition, for example, and the desire to echo the topography was used to establish the two distinct spaces. Instead of adding a porch to the room, Charlie had found a way to turn the room into a porch.

Rereading the letter, I realized he had achieved something much more difficult as well. My letter had articulated two completely contradictory images of the building: as a safe and wintry refuge on the one hand and, on the other, as a room that would throw itself open to the landscape. In Christopher Alexander's terms, these were the conflicting forces at work in my dream for the hut: the simultaneous desire for enclosure and freedom. Charlie had invented, or discovered, a form that promised to bring these two impulses into some kind of balance. Two thick walls holding up a thin roof: this was the pattern, more or less. And this pattern had been there almost from the beginning. Because there it was, right on the cover of Charlie's book of images, the design that had annoyed me with its obscurity and which now seemed clear as day:

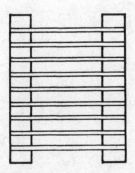

Using little more than this pair of thick walls, opened to the landscape on either end, Charlie had found a way to animate the space in the hut and grant his client's warring wishes for an equally strong sense of refuge and prospect.

On paper, at least. Because right now, any talk about the experience of space in my hut was idle, a matter of hunch and speculation. There was no way I could be sure Charlie's design worked the way he said it did without actually building it and moving in. This might not have been the case had Charlie designed a more conceptual or literary building—a hut built chiefly out of words or critical theories or signs, the kind that, once worked out on paper, is as good as built (if not better). Just think, this whole project would have been done now, everything but the explanatory texts. I could have slipped back into the warm tub of commentary, and never have had to learn how to cut a bird's mouth in a rafter or drill a half-inch hole through a boulder in order to pin it to a concrete pier. But no such luck. This particular building was meant to be experienced, not read. Only part of its story can be told on paper; the rest of it would be in wood.

CHAPTER 4

Footings

How to get your building down to the ground, the task that now confronted me, has always been a big issue for architects and builders, not only from an engineering perspective—the foundation being the place where a building is most vulnerable to the elements—but philosophically too.

This is perhaps especially true in America. Our architects seem to have devoted an inordinate amount of attention to the relationship of their buildings to the ground—which makes sense, in light of the fact that Americans have always believed, with varying degrees of conviction, that ours is somehow sacred ground, a promised land. The Puritans used to call the New World landscape "God's second book," and in the nineteenth century it became the preferred volume of the transcendentalists, who read the land for revelation and moral instruction. It is at any rate the ground of our freedom and, given our varied racial and ethnic composition, the one great thing we hold in common—the thing that makes us all Americans. So it matters how our buildings sit on this ground.

This might explain why, when you compare a great American house such as Monticello to the Palladian models on which it was based, the overriding impression is that Jefferson has put his house on much more sympathetic terms with the ground. Where Palladio's blocky, classical villas stand somewhat aloof from the earth, Monticello stretches out comfortably over its mountaintop site as if to complete, rather than dominate, it. The horizontal inflection that Jefferson gave to Monticello—this sense that a building should unfold along the ground—proved to be prophetic, for it eventually became one of the hallmarks of American architecture. It finds expression in the floor plans of turn-of-the-century shingle-style houses, which ramble almost like miniature landscapes in imitation of the ground on which they sit, and even in the ground-hugging ranch houses of postwar suburbia.

This same gesture of horizontal expansiveness, behind which surely stand dreams of the frontier and the open road, is what gave even a public work such as the Brooklyn Bridge its powerful sense of horizontal release—"Vaulting the sea," as Hart Crane wrote of it, and "the prairies' dreaming sod . . ." And though considerably darkened, the gesture survives in the Vietnam Veterans Memorial, in Washington, D.C., perhaps the most stirring meditation yet on the American ground. Along an extended horizontal slit cut into the Mall, the memorial draws us down into the American ground itself, where we come literally face to face with it, to contemplate at once its violation—the slab of granite chronicling the names of the dead it now holds—as well as its abiding power of healing and renewal.

But the greatest, and sunniest, poet of the American ground was Frank Lloyd Wright, who no doubt bore some responsibility for the complicated footings I was about to undertake as the construction of my hut began. Viewed from one perspective, Wright's lifelong project was to figure out how Americans might best make themselves at home on the land that forms this nation. "I had an idea," he wrote, "that the planes parallel to the earth in buildings identify themselves with the ground, do most to make the buildings belong to the ground." That this was something to be wished for went without saying for Wright, who liked to describe himself as "an American, child of the ground and of space."

"What was the matter with the typical American house?" he asked in a 1954 book called *The Natural House.* "Well just for an honest beginning, it lied about everything." It had no "sense of space as should belong to a free people" and no "sense of earth." The first defect he sought to remedy with his open, outward-thrusting floor plans and powerful horizontal lines. The second meant rethinking the foundation, something on which no architect before or since has lavished quite so much attention. (Though with my hut's footings, Charlie seemed to be mounting a respectable challenge.) Wright held that houses "should begin *on* the ground, not *in* it as they then began, with damp cellars." He spoke of conventional foundations and basements as if they were unpardonable violations of the sacred ground plane. Along with attics, basements also offended Wright's sense of democracy, since they implied a social hierarchy. (This was more than just a metaphor: Servants typically occupied one space or the other.) For Wright, the proper space of democracy was horizontal.

Wright devised several alternatives to the traditional foundation, including what he called the "dry wall footing": essentially a concrete slab at ground level set on a bed of gravel. But even when Wright built more conventional foundations, he would specify that the framing begin on the inside edge of the masonry wall rather than at the outer edge, as is the standard practice. The effect he was after was a kind of plinth, "a projecting base course" of masonry to help the house "*look* as though it began there *at* the ground." Not that this solution was really all that honest, since the house only *appeared* to rest on the ground; in fact, it often rested on a conventional foundation wall that sliced through the ground to form a cellar. Here where our buildings meet the earth, the ideal and the possible often seem to eye each other tensely.

Wright's projecting base course of stone also served visually to "weld the structure to the ground"—something, by the way, that at the time only an American was apt to deem desirable. For at the precise historical moment that Wright was taking such pains to wed his buildings to the land, many European modernists were turning their backs on it and dispensing with foundations altogether. Le Corbusier was setting his houses on slender white stilts, or "pilotis," that stepped gingerly over the ground as if it were unwholesome, touching it in as few places as possible and all but cursing the gravity that made contact with the earth necessary at all. The house of the future was supposed to be as rootless and streamlined as an airplane or ocean liner.

Even when Wright himself went to war against gravity, his purpose was not to escape the ground so much as to honor it. At Fallingwater, in western Pennsylvania, he cantilevered a house out over the waters of the Bear Run not so that it might seem to fly ("A house is not going anywhere," he once said, in a dig at Le Corbusier's vehicle worship, "at least not if we can help it"), but as a way to elaborate and extend the stratified rock ledge on which it is literally based. In a sense, Fallingwater is nothing *but* a foundation: The living space is a steel-reinforced concrete extension of the ledge rock that anchors the structure to the ground. Even a house as gravity-defying as this one was still what Wright said all American houses should be: "a sympathetic feature of the ground" expressing its "kinship to the terrain."

It was ideas such as these that stood behind Charlie's design for the footings of my hut, a sketch of which arrived in the mail in early October:

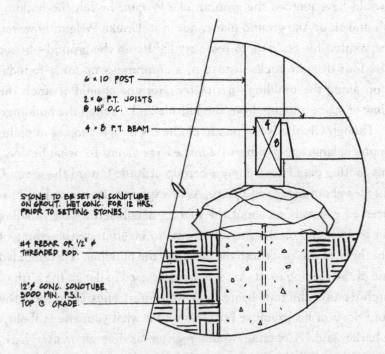

6 × 10 POST

2 × 6 P.T. JOISTS @ 16" O.C.

4 × 8 P.T. BEAM

STONE TO BE SET ON SONOTUBE ON GROUT. WET CONC. FOR 12 HRS. PRIOR TO SETTING STONES.

#4 REBAR OR 1/2" ø THREADED ROD.

12'ø CONC. SONOTUBE. 3000 MIN. P.S.I. TOP @ GRADE.

This somewhat daunting construction drawing made at least two things plain: A building's relationship to the ground was a more complicated matter than an architect might want it to appear, and the outward impression and the actual engineering of that relationship were two entirely different matters.

The impression Charlie sought to create with our rock footings (which he soon took to calling the building's "feet") was of an unusually comfortable, almost relaxed relationship between the hut and the ground. (In his original concept, you will recall, the building's relationship to the ground was *so* relaxed that I was going to need a house jack to square it up from time to time.) The four boulders on which the building sat (or at least appeared to sit) implied even more than a "kinship with the terrain"; they suggested the hut was in some sense part and parcel of its site.

Charlie's objection to standard concrete piers was that they would have pierced the ground; like Wright, he felt the building should sit on the ground plane, not in it. Unlike Wright, however, he wanted his building to rest very lightly on the ground—hence the four discrete rocks instead of a continuous masonry foundation along the building's perimeter. Nothing should staunch the flow of space coming down the hillside and through the building.

Though Charlie is not one to clothe his design choices in philosophical language or otherwise make large claims for what he does, his footing detail does imply a certain attitude toward the ground, an idea about nature and place. As he explained it to me when I expressed reservations about the footing detail, setting the building on rocks found on the site was a way "to incorporate something of the 'here' of this place into the design of the building." He reminded me of the etching Marc-Antoine Laugier used to depict the birth of architecture, the four living trees in a forest enlisted to form the four posts of his primitive hut. "Rocks are what your site is about," Charlie said. "Concrete would register as foreign matter here, something citified and imported. This is obviously not a primitive or vernacular building, but that doesn't mean it can't meet its place halfway, that there can't be some give and take."

Looked at from this perspective, any building represents a meeting place of the local landscape and the wider world, of what is given "Here" and what's been brought in from "There." The Here in this case is of course the site, but the site defined broadly enough to take in not only the sunlight and character of the ground, the climate and flora and slope, but also the local culture as it is reflected in the landscape—in the arrangements of field and forest and in the materials and styles commonly used to build "around here." Conceivably, a building could be based entirely on such local elements, but this happens more seldom than we think: Even a structure as seemingly indigenous as a log cabin built with local timber is based on an idea and a set of techniques imported in the eighteenth century from Scandinavia. Backwoods survivalist types living "off the grid," as they like to say, may flatter themselves about their independence, but in fact it is only the beavers and groundhogs who truly build locally, completely outside the influence of culture and history, beyond the long reach of There.

And There, of course, is just another way of saying the broader culture and economy, which in our time has become international. The term takes in everything from the prevailing styles of architecture and the state of technology to the various images and ideas afloat in the general culture, as well as such mundane things as the prime rate and the price of materials, labor, and energy. In fact a whole set of values can be grouped under the heading of "There," and these can be juxtaposed with a parallel set of values that fit under the rubric "Here":

THERE	HERE
Universal	Particular
Internationalism	Regionalism
Progress	Tradition
Classical	Vernacular
Idea	Fact
Information	Experience
Space	Place
Mobility	Stability
Palladio	Jefferson
Jefferson	Wright
Abstract	Concrete
Concrete	Rock

The juxtapositions can be piled up endlessly, and though matters soon get complicated (look what happens to concrete, or to Jefferson and Wright), they can still serve as a useful shorthand for two distinct ways of looking at, or organizing, the world.

The tension between the two terms is nothing new, of course. Thomas Jefferson was dealing with this when he imported Palladianism from Europe and gave it an American inflection; Monticello represents a novel synthesis of There and Here, of classicism and the American ground. (For Wright's taste and time, however, Jefferson was still too much the classicist, which suggests that Here and There are strictly relative.) In our own time, the balance between the two terms has been steadily tilting toward the There end of the scale. There are some powerful abstractions on the side of There, and in the last century or so these have tended to run over the local landscape. The force and logic of these abstractions are what have helped farmland to give way to tract housing, city neighborhoods to ambitious schemes of "urban renewal," and regional architecture to an "international style" that for a while elevated the principle of There—of universal culture—to a utopian program and moral precept. Modernism has always regarded Here as an anachronism, an impediment to progress. This might explain why so many of its houses walked the earth on white stilts, looking as though they wanted to get off, to escape the messy particularities of place for the streamlined abstraction of space.

One reason Frank Lloyd Wright was for many years regarded as old-fashioned (Philip Johnson, in his International Style days, famously dismissed Wright as "the greatest architect of the nineteenth century") is that, even as he set about inventing the space of modern architecture, he continued to insist on the importance of Here—of the American ground. Wright always upheld the value of a native and regional architecture (one for the prairie, another for the desert) and resisted universal culture in all its guises—whether it came dressed in the classicism of Thomas Jefferson, the internationalism of the Beaux Arts movement, or the modernism of Le Corbusier.

In retrospect, Wright's stance seems the more enlightened one, and these days everybody has a good word for regionalism and the sense of place. But it remains to be seen whether the balance between Here and There is actually being redressed, or whether universal culture, more powerful than ever, is merely donning a few quaint local costumes now that they're fashionable and benign. I've never visited a "neotraditional" town like Seaside, the planned community on the Florida panhandle celebrated for its humane postmodern architecture and sense of neighborhood, but I can't help wondering if the experience of sitting out on one of those great-looking front porches and chatting with the neighbors strolling by doesn't feel just a bit synthetic. In an age of Disney and cyberspace, it may not be possible to keep a crude pair of terms like Here and There straight too much longer, not when a "sense of place" becomes a commodity that can be bought and sold on the international market, and people blithely use homey metaphors of place to describe something as abstract and disembodied as the Internet.

=

So a lot more than wooden posts were resting on Charlie's rock feet. Intellectually, I had no problem with the footings, or what they stood for. One of the reasons I wanted to build this hut myself, after all, was to remedy the sense I had that I lived too much of my life in the realm of There, so steeped in its abstractions and mediations that Here had begun to feel like a foreign country. In a sense, Charlie's footing was exactly what I was looking for. What could be more Here, more real, than a rock?

And yet as his daunting sketch made plain, Charlie's rocks *weren't* entirely real. Oh, they were real enough in and of themselves, as I would soon find out trying to coax them to the site, but they couldn't really do what they appeared to do: hold up the corner posts that in turn held up the roof. The hidden concrete footing with the spike of steel running through it would have to do that. The rocks might be real, but the idea that they were holding up the building by themselves was nothing more than a romantic conceit, a metaphor.

That's because the building's supposedly "comfortable relationship" with the ground didn't take the reality of the ground into account. And the reality of the ground, American or otherwise, is that it doesn't particularly *want* a comfortable relationship with the buildings that sit on it, no matter who their architects are or how fond their regard for the land. Frank Lloyd Wright knew this, Charlie Myer knows this, anybody who's ever built knows this: The ground that really matters, the only ground on which we can safely found a building, lies several feet below the ground we honor, the precise depth depending on the downward extent of frost in any particular place.

Around here the figure is forty-two inches—which is simply the depth below which no one can recall the ground ever having frozen. Anywhere above this point, rocks and even boulders will be constantly on the move, gradually shouldering their way up toward the surface under the irresistible pressure of freezing and thawing water. And any rock that sits on top of the ground, however immobile it may appear, is liable to get up and dance during a January thaw. The evidence was all around this place: in the tumbled-down stone walls that bound these fields like smudged property lines, and in the wooded waste areas where the farmer dumped the new crop of boulders he hauled out of his fields each spring. The extraordinary prestige that the ground enjoys, reflected in so many of our metaphors of stability and truth, is largely undeserved: Sooner or later that ground will be betrayed by a shifting underground. Which is why, in latitudes where the earth freezes every winter, a comfortable-looking relationship to the ground will require a somewhat uncomfortable amount of architectural subterfuge.

I wasn't prepared to face up to the metaphysical implications of this fact quite yet, but I was ready to confront a practical one: If I was actually going to construct such a footing—one that implied a certain relationship to the ground but in fact depended on a very different (and undisclosed) relationship and therefore required not only the ostensible rock footing but a subtext of concrete and steel as well as a system to join these real and apparently real elements together—then I was going to need some help. I decided to take Judith's advice and hire somebody, not only to assist with the footings but also to guide me through the countless other complexities that I was beginning to suspect Charlie's "idiot-proof" design held in store.

Joe Benney was the man I had in mind. I first met Joe during the renovation of our house, when he was moonlighting for our contractor, helping out with the demolition, insulation, and all those other unglamorous construction tasks builders are only too happy to sub out. Joe's day job at the time was in a body shop; fixing up wrecked cars is his passion, though bodywork is by no means his only marketable skill. Joe is, at twenty-seven, a master of the material world, equally at home in the realms of steel, wood, soil, plants, concrete, and machinery. At various times he has made his living as a mechanic (working on cars, diesel engines, and hydraulic rigs), a carpenter, a tree surgeon, a house painter, an excavator, a landscaper, a welder, and a footing man on a foundation crew. He also knows his way around plumbing and gardens and guns.

As you might guess from the number of careers Joe has already had at twenty-seven, none of them have lasted very long. From what I've gathered, and observed, the problem, if it is one, has to do with Joe's mouth, not his hands. Joe hasn't much patience for the kind of boss who fails to acknowledge that Joe knows more about his business than he does, which, unfortunately for Joe, happens to be the great majority of bosses. As I would soon find out for myself, Joe can also be a bit of a hothead; he says it's his Irish blood. These qualities make for frequent job shifts and periods of unemployment, though since he is so variously talented these never last very long.

It happened that at the time I was puzzling over Charlie's footing drawing, Joe was looking for some weekend work. I told him about the building, which I had been hoping to work on on weekends, and he offered to swing by to talk about it. Joe drives a small, somewhat beat-up Mitsubishi pickup, a vehicle longer on character than inspection-worthiness: no bumpers to speak of, smashed taillights, Grateful Dead decals on the cab window, and the name of his daughter—Shannon Marie—painted across the front of the hood. If not for the signature vehicle, I might not have recognized the fellow who climbed out of it that afternoon, with the broad cascade of auburn curls reaching halfway down his back. It's only on a day off that you'll see Joe without the cap (woolen in winter, baseball in summer) that he tucks his ponytail up into, to keep it clean on the job and perhaps also to keep down the grief. Joe is not very tall, but he's a powerfully built thumb of a man, and depending on the current line of work, one section or another of his body is apt to be stuffed with muscle. Leaving aside his expertise, I very much liked the idea of having someone as strong as Joe around to help move boulders and lift six-by-ten posts.

We walked out to the site, where I showed him Charlie's sketches for the building as well as the footing detail. He studied the drawings for a minute or two, made the obligatory carpenter's crack about architects ("ivory tower," etc.), and then said what he always says any time you ask him if he might be interested in a project:

"Piece a cake."

We settled on an hourly rate and agreed to get started as soon as I had my building permit and the holes for the footing could be dug. Originally I had planned on digging them myself, but a backhoe was going to be on the property later in the month (to repair the pond; it's a long story), so I'd figured I might as well have the excavator do it. Digging a half-dozen four-foot-deep holes in this ground by hand was a job I was happy to skip; it's one thing to honor the rocks around here, and quite another to confront them at the end of a spade. Before he took off, Joe offered to give me a hand staking out each of the six holes to be dug—one at each of the building's corners and then a pair in the middle of the rectangle, where the building would step down with the grade of the site.

Charlie and I had already staked two of the corners over the July Fourth weekend, deciding on the building's precise location with respect to the rock (crouching a few steps back so as not to upstage it) as well as its orientation to the sun. Joe asked me how we'd determined the precise angle. It hadn't been easy. The obvious solution would have been to adopt the orientation of the small clearing alongside the boulder, which ran more or less due east to west. But that angle would have admitted too much direct sunlight through the front window of the building, even with its visor, particularly on spring and autumn afternoons. Due west also put the big ash tree directly in my line of sight, which promised to block the sense of prospect from the desk.

So Charlie and I had experimented, the two of us standing side by side where the front window would be, facing dead straight ahead and revolving our bodies in a stiff, incremental pirouette, one of us occasionally leaving the front line to check the view from another imaginary window. As we pivoted the building on its axis, each ten-degree shift in angle caused a revolution in perspective from every window. We would nudge the front of the building into a winning prospect only to find that the south-facing casement window now stared out at a Ford Pinto up on blocks in my neighbor's yard. This must have gone on for an hour or more, both of us reluctant to give up without testing every conceivable angle. We were planting the building, after all, determining what was going to be my angle on things for a long time to come. Finally we hit upon one that seemed to satisfy all the windows and avoid a too-direct confrontation with the ash or the afternoon sun. By the compass, my angle on things was going to be 255 degrees, or 15 degrees south of due west.

Now Joe and I made preparations to fix this perspective in concrete. Once we had planted the four corner stakes, making sure they formed a rectangle of the dimensions specified on Charlie's footing plan (14'2" by 8'9"), we checked to make sure it was square by measuring the diagonals; if the lengths of the two diagonals were equal, that meant the rectangle was square. This may have been the first time in my life I had successfully applied an axiom learned in high school geometry. Though I didn't fully appreciate it at the time, I was opening a chapter in my life in which the rules of geometry would loom as large as the rules of grammar ordinarily do. It seemed like a snap, too, but then I still had no idea how much less forgiving the new rules could be.

Now we had a life-size diagram of the building, outlined on the ground in yellow nylon string, and the effect of it, on the site but also on my spirits, was larger than I might have guessed. Part of it, I suppose, was the sense of satisfaction that often comes from making a straight line in nature—whether in a row of seedlings, a garden path, or a baseball diamond. "Geometry is man's language," Le Corbusier used to say, and it was cheering to see this perfect rectangle take shape on the rough, unreliable ground. (Who knows, but the fact that the rectangle's proportions chimed with the Golden Section might have had something to do with it too.) All our abstract drawings on paper were at last being transferred to the real world.

While I stood there admiring the view from inside my box of string, Joe had been sitting up on top of the big rock, studying Charlie's footing plan. He had been uncommonly quiet up to now, merely nodding as I explained to him the thinking behind the various decisions Charlie and I had made, and I had taken his silence for consensus. More likely, he'd been doing his best not to second-guess us, because now he interrupted my reverie with a question.

"Do you really want to put fir posts directly on top of a rock?"

I didn't see why not.

"In one word? Rot."

He explained that the end grain of the posts would wick up moisture from the boulders they sat on, a bad enough situation made worse by the fact that, among woods, fir offers relatively little resistance to rot.

"My building, I'd do it differently. But it's up to you."

"It's up to you" just might be the single most irritating thing you can say to somebody under the circumstances, a cranky parody of the liberty it pretends to bestow. But I decided to keep a lid on my annoyance.

"So how do you suggest we do it?"

"Couple of options," he began, settling a little too quickly into the role of tutor, his laconic manner of a few moments ago now a memory. I was treated to a detailed lecture about the virtues and drawbacks of pressure-treated lumber (wood that has been immersed under pressure in a solution of chemicals, including arsenic and copper, to kill off the microorganisms that dine on wood). This was followed by a disquisition on the relative weather-resistance of a dozen different tree species, beginning with pine (highly vulnerable) and ending with locust, which is so hard and rot resistant that it can be sunk naked into the ground. Redwood or cedar would apparently last much longer than fir, though both were considerably more expensive. Finally, Joe ran through a list of the various wood preservatives and sealants on the market, things we could apply to the end grain if I decided to stick with fir.

Everything Joe was saying sounded sensible, but I told him I wanted to consult with Charlie before making a decision. This was the wrong thing to say. I should simply have said I wanted to think it over. Invoking Charlie's authority clearly annoyed Joe, who evidently had already concluded that Charlie was just another ivory-tower architect with his head in the clouds, if not someplace worse. Joe works hard at seeming to take things in stride, however. He maintains a whole vocabulary of phrases to indicate how nonchalant he is—"piece a cake," "cool," "I'm easy," "no problem," "no sweat"—as well as some novel contractions of these, one of which he now produced, along with a slightly offended, suit-yourself hike of the shoulders:

"Cake."

Joe's monosyllabic shrug masked strong feelings, and immediately I could see that this construction project was not going to escape the edginess that traditionally crops up between architects and builders, a complicated set of tensions rooted in real differences of outlook and interest and, inevitably, social class. On building sites all over the world, architects are figures of ridicule, their designs derided for their oddness or impracticality and their construction drawings, which on a job site are supposed to have the force of law, dismissed as cartoons or "funny papers." What remained to be seen on this particular site, however, was exactly where I fit into this drama, since I was both client (traditionally an ally of the architect) and builder. The fact that I would be working on this project, and not just paying for it, changed everything. I was the patron of Charlie's fancy ideas, but I also faced the practical problem of making them work, something I probably couldn't manage without Joe's help. Among other things, Joe was poking around to see whose authority I was placing first.

And I wasn't sure. Joe had shifted the ground on me a bit, which is why I hoped to table for the time being the issue of how our fir posts would meet their rock feet. I'd always regarded Charlie as a realist among architects, somebody with his own feet planted firmly in the world, and an authority on practical questions. His footing detail may have gotten a little baroque, but that was only because its romance of the ground had been tempered by what seemed like some hardheaded realism about it—hence the four feet of concrete and the steel rods. What could possibly be more down-to-earth than that footing drawing?

But if Joe was right, he had spotted what appeared to be the Achilles' heel of Charlie's footing detail. It wasn't a problem we had to solve right away—whatever we did about it, the concrete piers first had to be poured, the boulders drilled and pinned. Touchy though he might be at times, I felt relieved to know Joe would be along on what promised to be a treacherous voyage to the material underworld. I'd found my prickly Virgil.

≡

A few weeks later I paid a visit to Bill Jenks, the local building inspector. Though Charlie hadn't quite finished the construction drawings, with his rough sketches and the footing plan I could apply for the building permit I would need before Joe and I could pour the footings. On any construction project, the building inspector is a slightly intimidating figure, since he wields the power to order expensive changes in a design or force a builder to redo any work that isn't "up to code." He is the final authority—the building trade's judge, superego, and reality principle rolled into one—and he holds the power to condemn any building that doesn't meet his approval. I once asked a contractor whom he appealed to when there was a difference of opinion with the building inspector. The fellow squinted at me for the longest time, trying to determine if I could possibly be serious. He'd never heard of anyone questioning a ruling from the building inspector. But surely there must be *some* court of appeal, I insisted. What about due process? The Fourteenth Amendment? "I suppose you could appeal to the governor," he offered after long reflection. "Weicker *might* be able to overrule Jenks."

"Code" consists of a few thousand rules, most of them commonsensical (the minimum dimension of a doorway, for example: 2′4″) but many others obscure and seemingly picayune (the maximum number of gallons of water in a toilet tank: 1.6). The house that satisfies every jot and tittle of the building code probably hasn't been built yet, which is why a building inspector is given wide latitude in the exercise of his judgments. He has the authority to sign off on minor transgressions. Or he can go strictly by the book. Most of the contractors I've met live in constant low-grade terror of the building inspector.

You might think that, since the building inspector's mission in life is to look out for the interests of the consumer, who on this particular job happened to be me, Jenks could in this instance be expected to go fairly easy. In the days before my interview with him, the approach of which instilled in me a moderate but unshakable level of dread, I'd taken no small comfort in this theory. But when I tried it out on Joe, the night before my meeting, he said I could forget it. The building inspector is paid to take a very, very long view, Joe explained. He's thinking about hundred-year storms (the worst storm to hit a region in a century, a conventional standard for structural strength) and about the persons yet unborn who will own and occupy my hut in the next century.

My first impression of Jenks did little to relieve my anxiety. Actually, it wasn't an impression of Jenks himself, but of his boots, which stood rigidly at attention outside the door to his office. They were knee-high black riding boots, easily a size thirteen, that had been arrayed with military precision and buffed to a parade-ground sheen. The boots said two things to me, neither of them reassuring. First, any man who would wear them was without a doubt drunk with power, very possibly a closet sadist or a collector of Nazi paraphernalia. Second, such a person had a serious fetish for meticulousness: You could shave in the shine on these boots, they butted the wall at ninety degrees dead on, and the space between them appeared to have been microcalibrated.

These were the boots of the man who would be judging my craftsmanship each step of the way.

Fortunately, the man himself wasn't quite as intimidating as his footwear, though he certainly took his sweet time looking over the drawings I spread out across his drafting table. Jenks was slender and tall, perhaps six foot two, though his posture made him seem considerably taller: The man was plumb. Picture a two-by-four with a handlebar mustache. For a long time Jenks said nothing, just stood there smoothing down the ends of his great black handlebars as he walked his eyes over every inch of Charlie's drawings.

"Looks to be sturdy enough," he announced at last. I took this as a compliment, until I realized he was making fun of the beefy four-by fir timbers Charlie had spec'd for the frame, which were substantially more substantial than a one-story outbuilding required. "See a lot of tornadoes out your way?" I laughed, largely, and it seemed as though everything was going to be all right. Which it was, until he got to the footing detail and stopped. He began tapping the drawing with his pencil eraser, lightly at first, then much harder and faster. "Nope. I won't approve this as drawn. Any framing within eight inches of the ground must be pressure-treated, and that includes the posts sitting on these rocks." Joe had been right; the footing was indeed my hut's Achilles' heel.

But Jenks was willing to give me the building permit anyway, provided I signed a piece of paper promising to make the changes he specified. He instructed me to call for a field inspection as soon as we'd poured the footing, then again when the framing was complete. I left his office feeling buoyant, official, launched at last. When I got home I walked out to the site and nailed the bright yellow cardboard building permit to a tree. The following morning, we would pour.

≡

Concrete is peculiar stuff, so accommodating one moment, so adamant the next. Not that it's the least bit mercurial—few things in this world are as reliable as concrete. Wet, it can be counted on to do almost anything you want; it's as happy taking its formal cues from a mold as it is acceding to gravity. Vertical, horizontal, square or curved, ovoid or triangular, concrete can be made to do it all, no complaints. Once cured, however, the stuff's incorrigible, as stubborn and implacable as rock. What was feckless is now transcendently determined, and all but immortal. In the case of concrete, there's no turning back, no melting it down to try again, as plastic or metal permits, no cutting it to fit, like wood. Here in a handful of cold gray glop is the irreversible arrow of time, history's objective correlative. A fresh batch of concrete can pass into the future along an almost infinite number of paths—as road, bridge, pier, sculpture, building, or bench—but once a path is taken, it is as one-way and fixed as fate. Right here is where the two meanings of the word "concrete"—the thing and the quality—intersect: for what else in the world is more *particular?*

These are the kinds of thoughts working with concrete inspires, on a suitably gray and chilly November afternoon. Although one or two steps in the process are critical, for the most part mixing and pouring concrete doesn't fully engage the intellect, leaving plenty of room for daydream or reflection. Mainly it's your back that's engaged, hauling the eighty-pound sacks of ready-mix to the site, pouring them into a wheelbarrow along with twelve quarts of water per bag, and then mixing the stiff, bulky batter with a rake until it's entirely free of lumps. The stuff is very much like a cake mix, in fact, except that each batch weighs more than three hundred pounds (three bags plus nine gallons of water) and licking the fork is not a temptation. You can make concrete from scratch too, mixing the gravel, sand, and Portland cement (a powder fine as flour) according to the standard recipe (roughly, 3:2:1 for a foundation), but for a job this size Joe had recommended ready-mix, the Betty Crocker of concrete.

Pliny wrote somewhere that apples were the heaviest of all things. I don't know about that. It's my impression that eighty pounds of concrete weighs a good deal more than eighty pounds of almost anything else, apples included. Apples at least show some inclination toward movement—they will roll, given half a chance—whereas a bag of concrete lying on the ground very much wants to stay there. Add water, and the resultant mud is so thick and heavy—so stubbornly inert—that dragging a tool through it even once is a project. I would plunge my rake head down into the mire and then pull at it with all the strength I could summon, which yielded maybe six or seven inches of movement, copious grunts, and an almost exquisite frustration at the sheer indifference of matter at rest. Hats off, I thought, to the Mafia capo who first perceived the unique possibilities for horror in sinking a man's feet in cement. For Joe the stuff behaved a good deal more like cake batter, however, and whenever my stirring grew so lugubrious that the concrete threatened to set, he would take the rake from me and, throwing his powerful back and shoulders into the work, whip the concrete smooth as if with a wire whisk.

For forms we were using sonotubes, which are nothing more than thick cardboard cylinders—stiffened, oversize toilet paper rolls sunk into the earth. Whenever Joe judged a batch of concrete "good to go," the two of us would shoulder the wheelbarrow into position, tip it down toward the lip of the sonotube and then, with a shovel, herd the cold gray slurry into the cylinder. It would land four feet down at the bottom of the shaft with a sequence of satisfying plops. The sonotubes were cavernous—fourteen inches in diameter, broad enough to give our boulders a nice, comfortable seat—and it took almost two barrow loads to fill each one. But by the end of the day all six had been filled—more than a ton of concrete mixed and poured by hand. Then with a hacksaw we cut lengths of threaded steel rod and inserted them in the center of each concrete cylinder. We bent the submerged end of each rod to improve its purchase on the concrete and then left about eight inches exposed above the top of the pier; to this pin we would bolt our boulders.

By now the two of us matched the color of the dimming, overcast sky, each cloaked in a fine gray powder that had infiltrated every layer of our clothing, even our skin. I don't think my hands have ever been more dry; the insides of my nose and sinuses felt like they were on fire. (Joe said that the limestone in the Portland cement sucked the moisture out of tissue.) I was also exhausted, stiff, and chilled to the bone, wet concrete being not only heavier than any known substance, but colder too. Some part of me that didn't appreciate these sensations inquired sarcastically if the experience had been sufficiently real. Joe counseled a hot shower, ibuprofen, and a tube of Ben-Gay.

≡

By the next morning the concrete had cured enough that I could stand on the piers. To do so was to acquire a whole new appreciation of the concept of stability. Maybe it was just the hardness of the concrete, or the width of the piers, which were as big around as the seat of a chair, but I had a powerful sense that I stood upon reliable ground, beyond the reach of frost heaves or flood, beyond, in fact, the reach of almost any vicissitude I could think of. Suddenly I understood the prestige and authority of foundations. Whatever happens to the building erected on top of it, bound as it is to bend under the pressures of weather and time and taste, the foundation below will endure. The woods all around here are littered with them, ancient cellar holes lined in fieldstone. Though the frame houses they once supported have vanished without trace, the foundations remain, crusted with lichens but otherwise unperturbed.

I could see why so many writers and philosophers would be drawn to the authority of foundations for their metaphors of permanence and transcendence. The classic example is *Walden*, which is at bottom (to borrow one of the book's most well-worn metaphors) an extended search for a good foundation—for the ground on which to build a better, truer life. Thoreau's goal, he tells us in "Where I Lived, and What I Lived For," is to reach down "below freshet and frost and fire [to] a place where you might found a wall or a state, or set a lamppost safely, or perhaps a gauge, not a Nilometer, but a Realometer, that future ages might know how deep a freshet of shams and appearances had gathered from time to time." Truth is to be found below the frost line.

Western philosophers have always been attracted to such images of the reliable ground, along with the various other architectural metaphors that arise from it. Descartes depicted philosophy as the building of a structure on a well-grounded foundation; in similar language, Kant described metaphysics as an "edifice" of thought raised up on secure "foundations" that in turn must be placed on stable "ground." Heidegger, a critic of this tradition (who nevertheless likened thinking to building), defined metaphysics as a search for "that upon which everything rests"—a search for a reliable foundation. By borrowing these kinds of metaphors, philosophers have sought to grant some of the firmness, logic, and objectivity of buildings to systems of thought that might otherwise seem a good deal less manifest or authoritative. Architectural metaphors can also lend an air of immortality to a philosophical idea, perhaps because there are buildings standing in Europe that are older than philosophy itself.

So it makes good sense that contemporary critics of metaphysics—who, tellingly, lump all of its various schools and practitioners under the rubric of "foundationalism"—would spend as much time and energy as they do attacking its reliance on architectural metaphors. Jacques Derrida has made a brilliant career of illuminating the inconstant "undergrounds" beneath the supposedly firm and final ground of metaphysical truth. It's for good reason that the most famous critique of metaphysics goes by the name of "deconstruction." (There is a large irony here in the fact that, after centuries of lending philosophers the authority of their architectural metaphors, architects today should be so eager to borrow the one metaphor from philosophy—deconstruction—whose express purpose is to attack that very authority.)

But while the prestige of foundations may have been unfairly exploited over the years in the selling of various philosophical and literary bills of goods, it's hard to see why this borrowing should make anyone doubt the credibility of unmetaphorical foundations—the kind made out of real concrete and steel. Whether or not Thoreau can fairly lay claim to it, whether or not I can actually sense it standing on top of my concrete piers, a certain kind of truth *does* reside forty-two inches beneath the ground, down there beneath freshet and frost. A foundation rooted this deeply can be counted on in a way that, say, some philosopher's idea of the truth cannot, no matter how "grounded" he claims it to be. For one thing, I don't have to subscribe to its meaning in order for it to work. It *doesn't* mean; it just is—something hard and real and unambiguous that Joe and I have added to the world. Step down on the footing, hard, and you will not think: *Hmmm . . . ambiguous.*

But what about the building that doesn't have such a good foundation to stand on? What happens when builders dispense with their notions of frost-line truth in the way that some contemporary philosophers have? While Joe and I were humping progressively more obstinate sacks of concrete from his truck out to the site, I'd speculated out loud about whether it was absolutely essential for a footing to go the full forty-two inches. I knew all about frost heaves, but I was starting to wonder just how big a difference it would really make, aside from the inconvenience of sticking doors and windows, if my building did move a few inches this way or that each winter—if it went along with the natural slipping and sliding of earth, rather than trying to resist it absolutely. Exhaustion can sometimes encourage one's thoughts in a romantic or even relativistic direction, and with each sack of mud mix I hoisted to my shoulder, the notion of building directly on boulders, of letting the ground have its way with the building, seemed a little less crazy, and even sort of poetic. If things got too far out of kilter, I could always resort to the house jack.

Joe, who can carry two bags of ready-mix at a time, one on each shoulder, had offered me a quick refresher from high school geometry about the instability of four-sided forms as compared to, say, three-sided ones. It's a fairly easy matter to collapse a cube by applying pressure to its surfaces unevenly, which accounts for the ubiquity of tripods, the endurance of pyramids. But long before our cube would collapse, the shifting of its foundation would set in motion an incremental process that would doom the building just as surely. The slightest movement of the footings would ramify throughout the structure, gradually eroding one after another of its right angles; "trueness," in the carpenter's sense, is the first casualty of a poor foundation. First the door frame falls out of square, since it is braced on only three sides. Then the windows. A building is a brittle thing, and eventually its seal against the weather will be broken—through a crack in the roof, perhaps, or in the slight discrepancy that arises between a ninety-degree window sash and what has become an eighty-nine-degree window frame. Now, a drip at a time, water enters the building and the process of its decomposition begins. As Joe put it, "Pretty soon, it's termite food."

As it happened, the dismal end result of precisely this process could be observed only a few steps from the sturdy pier on which I stood. In the woods on the far side of the path to the site stood, or I should say *lay*, a pair of decrepit outbuildings that had recently collapsed. Today these structures are nothing more than a sandwich of boards, but ten years ago, when we bought the place, a wall or two still stood—they were still recognizable as *buildings*. I remember thinking that they looked like capsized boats arrested in the process of sinking, in slow motion, back into the land. One of the structures appeared to have been a handyman's shack, the other a chicken coop. The ridge beam of the shack had collapsed on one side, submerging one end of the house in underbrush. The floor by now was earth, the floorboards having rotted away, and a maple tree was growing out through the window at the gable end still standing. Inside, if that word still meant anything, staghorn sumacs were ganged around a rusted stove.

It was a forlorn, slightly spooky place. Fewer than twenty years had passed since someone had lived here, and already the signs of habitation had grown faint, as the forest went methodically about the business of erasing the shack from the landscape. Lumber was reverting to trees, geometry to rank growth, and inside to outside, in a swift reversal of human work. Today, all that remains is a roughly shuffled deck of boards sprawled amid the second growth, something you might not notice if it wasn't pointed out.

I don't know for a fact that a shallow footing is responsible for the shack's ruin. It could as easily have started with a leak in the roof. But however it found its way in, the culprit, the chief means by which the forest reclaims any human construction, is the same: water. Lumber may not be alive exactly, but it is still part of the nutrient cycle of the forest and will return to it sooner or later. With our foundations and shingles, our paint and caulk and weather strip, we can stave off that time, postpone wood's fate, sometimes for hundreds of years. But, like everything else once alive, lumber is on loan from the land and in thrall to water, which, in concert with the conspiracy of insects and microorganisms we call rot, eventually will reduce it to compost. In the end it was this tug of life that pulled down the shack.

It occurred to me that, on my little chart, the ruined shack definitely came under the heading of "Here," and now even more than during its inhabited days. Indeed, the shack was in the process of succumbing utterly to the Here of this place; it was precisely those elements that had come from There—the geometry of its rafters; the manufactured goods on its shelves; the electrical wiring that, by linking the shack to the national grid, had made it possible to read a book or write a letter in it after dark—that nature was erasing. It is Here, I realized, that abhors all those things and has as its purpose their obliteration. In its ultimate form, Here consisted not only of the local boulders we planned to enlist in the new building's footings, but also the local termites and bacteria and the dark sift of compost forming on the forest floor beneath the old building, all the cycles of growth and decay at work in this ground, its powerful tug of life—and also death. (Which is one unromantic fact about the ground that the Vietnam Veterans Memorial does not overlook.) No, Here wasn't necessarily something you wanted to embrace too tightly.

It was in fact something you wanted to thwart, to defy, even as you flattered it with romantic architectural details such as rock footings. "Nature is hard to overcome," we read in *Walden*, of all places, "but she must be overcome." This, according to Le Corbusier, is architecture's first principle and purpose: to defy time and decay. That, and to wrest a space from nature to house all those things we value—books, conversation, marriage—that nature has no place or use for. A good foundation, these three and a half feet of concrete interposed between me and the damp, hungry ground, is how we start.

≡

Yet it is only a start. For even with the three and a half feet of concrete, Joe and Jenks were both convinced my foundation would fail my building unless something was done about the joining of its wood frame to its rock feet. When I first brought this problem to Charlie's attention, soon after Joe raised it, he had suggested we could simply soak the end grain of the fir in a bucket of Cuprinol, no big deal. Later, when I told him Jenks was insisting on pressure-treated posts, Charlie seemed taken aback, and somewhat resistant. Charlie knew perfectly well that code prohibited untreated wood to come within eight inches of the ground; he had just figured the boulders themselves would provide that margin. It was a question of perspective: To Charlie the boulders were part of the foundation; to Jenks they were part of the ground.

Charlie hated the idea of going to pressure-treated. The corner posts figured prominently in his design, and pressure-treated lumber is ugly stuff. Most of the wood used in the process is inferior to start with, typically an unlovely species like Southern yellow pine, which has a tendency to "check," or crack, along its loose, uneven grain. The chemical bath in which the wood is soaked also tinges it an artificial shade of green that is virtually impossible to remove or hide. I asked him about switching to redwood or cedar, as Joe had suggested. He guessed the cost would be prohibitive (and he was right: six-by-ten redwood posts would have cost $280 each, cedar not a whole lot less), and anyway, those species seemed too exotic for my hut. Fir might come from the Northwest, Charlie said, but it was used so commonly in New England as to be a vernacular building material. Another Here/There deal, in other words. I didn't think I wanted to mention this line of logic to Joe.

Charlie said he needed a few days to come up with an alternative. In the meantime, Joe and I moved ahead with the footings. We spent part of one Sunday collecting eligible boulders from around the property. Not surprisingly, the land offered a rich field of candidates, and we carefully weighed the dimensions, color, and geology of several dozen, factoring in a handicap based on a given boulder's proximity to the site. A cubic foot of granite weighs approximately 150 pounds, so a boulder sitting more than, say, a hundred yards from the foundation really had to be gorgeous to receive serious consideration. Within an hour we had wheelbarrowed or rolled a half-dozen promising rocks to the site, most of them flattish specimens of granite or gneiss about a yard wide and at least eighteen inches deep; anything smaller, we decided, would seem dinky beneath the big posts. We avoided shale or slate, rock that is more likely to crack under pressure, and even though we found some nice limestone and marble, these didn't *look* indigenous, so we passed. In short order I'd become a connoisseur of the local stone and could see that Cornwall rock had a certain look to it. Its skin was mottled gray-green, and its shapes were softly rounded, every sharpness weathered away. So these qualities became part of our ideal.

Joe had managed to borrow a rotary hammer from a landscaper he worked for, and the tool, which is actually a high-powered drill, made surprisingly easy work of boring half-inch holes through the boulders for our pins. The drill was the size of a viola and heavy enough that it wanted two hands, and ideally a big gut, to hold it steady, like a jackhammer. We took turns, one of us wielding the drill, the other a bucket of water, used to dissipate the heat generated by the bit boring through rock and to flush out the fine stone dust that collected in the deepening cavity. The bit emitted a terrible scream as it ate into the stone, but the granite yielded easily, almost as if it were tooth.

Now the boulders looked like monstrous gemstones; strung on a length of steel cable, they'd make a necklace for a Cyclops. We set them in mortar, slopping scoops of steel gray mud on top of the piers to form a custom-fitted seat beneath each rock. It took the two of us to hoist a boulder over its steel rod, struggling to line up the tiny hole with the even tinier pin, a process not unlike threading a 350-pound needle. The weight of the rocks could easily have crumpled the steel, so before we could begin to lower a boulder onto its pin we had to position the opening over it exactly, peering through the pinhole in the rock, as if it were the lens of a microscope, until the tiny metallic point swam into view. As we struggled to reconcile these rough beasts to their improbable new purpose, the orderly drafting table in Cambridge where the rock footings had had their immaculate conception seemed a world or two away. Did Charlie have any idea what was involved in making these footings actually work? For the first (but not the last) time, I was able to join in Joe's diatribe against the architectural profession with some gusto.

After we'd secured our boulders to their pins with lug nuts, two more holes in each rock remained to be drilled, to anchor the pins that would hold the posts in place, preventing any sideways movement, or "shear." Now the location of each hole became more critical still, so we measured our diagonals once again to make sure we were square. Next we cut a short length of steel rod for each hole, into which we squeezed a dab of Rockite, a space-age mortar that Joe claimed would form a bond stronger even than the granite itself; once the stuff set, it supposedly could hold up a truck. The other end of each rod we'd slip into a hole drilled in the bottom of a post.

Now our footings were ready to receive their posts—once we'd settled, that is, on an acceptable way to join them. Charlie had come back with the idea of using post anchors: small aluminum platforms that are typically used to protect the wood framing on decks from their concrete footings. A post anchor is like a shoe; it elevates the wood an inch or so above the concrete in order to keep its end grain from getting wet. Since post anchors are commonly used to join ordinary lumber to concrete, we figured the precedent might help persuade Jenks to accept Charlie's footing paradigm— in which the boulders are regarded as part of the foundation rather than the ground—and drop his insistence on pressure-treated lumber. The only problem was, we could find no manufacturer who made post anchors large enough to accommodate a six-by-ten post. The biggest we could find were six by six.

First Charlie suggested we have anchors custom made, a notion I refused to pay the respect of serious consideration. I'd already been floored by the quotes I was getting from lumberyards for the "appearance grade" fir Charlie had spec'd for my posts ($80 each; I needed eight), and I told him I wasn't about to engage the services of a metal foundry in the construction of a hut. A day or two later he faxed me a sketch, in which he proposed we cut back the ends of our posts at an angle so they could accommodate six-by-six post anchors, like so:

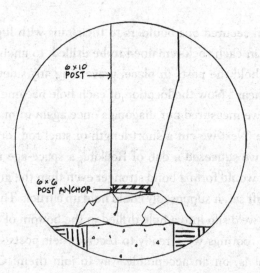

A note was scribbled beneath the drawing: "How about high-heeled shoes for our posts, instead of workboots? I kind of like it." I didn't. They looked like pigs' feet to me, incongruously feminine, and far too delicate for the weight they had to bear. It seemed to me the footings were getting too fancy now, too *careful*. They made you think of furniture, the legs of which traditionally taper as they near the ground in a gesture of refinement. In a building, which I think of as being a lot more businesslike about how it gets its weight down to the ground, the same gesture seemed too clever, even slightly ironic.

Then I had an idea of my own. Why couldn't we simply place a thin piece of pressure-treated lumber between the end grain of the post and the surface of the rock? If this wooden pad had the same footprint as the posts—a ten-inch section of a two-by-six, say—it would scarcely be visible, especially after the wood had aged. We could sell it to Jenks on the theory that it was no different from the pressure-treated sills builders commonly interpose between ordinary wood framing and the top of a new foundation. Aside from the fact that nobody else had come up with the idea, which made me suspect some lurking flaw in it, my pressure-treated minisill seemed like a workable and cheap solution. So what had I overlooked?

First I tried the idea out on Joe, who loved it. He even broke out one of his cherished workplace clichés for the occasion: "Mike, you're a genius with a *J*." And I did sort of feel like patting myself on the back, this being very possibly the most nuts-and-bolts empirical idea I had had in my life. Charlie was considerably less enthusiastic, however. My solution would work all right, he allowed, but it was inelegant.

"Come on, Charlie, we're talking about a *tiny* detail here. Nobody is ever going to notice it, except maybe you."

"I can't help it," he grumped. "I'm a micro-architect. These 'tiny' details are everything."

But Charlie understood the time had come to compromise. He had to concede my solution was a whole lot better than pressure-treated posts, and he offered to call Jenks to make the case as to why the boulders should be regarded as part of the foundation and my pressure-treated shoes as traditional foundation sills.

Jenks bought it. We were off the ground at last.

≡

Three and a half feet of concrete, three threaded steel rods, a few scoops of mortar, one granite boulder, one lug nut, two dabs of Rockite, and now a pair of pressure-treated shoes: my hut's "rustic" rock footing had certainly gotten complicated since Charlie first conceived it. As Joe and I worked on the pressure-treated pads, drilling and then seating them on their own beds of mortar, I thought about just how much effort, ingenuity, and technology it had taken to achieve such a seemingly simple and artless effect. Yet to look at the footings now was to have no idea of their complexity: Here were four boulders in a clearing in the woods, laid out to form a rectangle. Aside from the wooden pads sitting on them, the only clue to the fact that these were no ordinary boulders were the incongruous silver lug nuts that bolted them to the world.

And yet the footings weren't perfect, at least by their architect's lights. Until now, all of the artifice and subterfuge employed in their construction had been invisible, kept backstage or underground. But the pressure-treated shoes promised to alter slightly the hut's appearance, to put a tiny crimp in the "comfortable relationship" between its corner posts and the ground. Its posts would be barefoot no longer. Their new shoes constituted the building's first visible compromise with the exigencies of construction—the hut's first declension from its drafting-table ideal.

This bothered me at first. But after a while I began to appreciate that such compromises were an inevitable part of the work of building, if not, in some sense, its very essence. The building that refuses to embrace the contingencies of regulation and economics, of the weather and the ground, of the available technology and the abilities of its builders, is a building that never gets built. Joe has an expression he trots out from time to time, often around quitting time, when we've paused to look over the day's work, or after he's decided that some bit of carpentry he's been struggling with for too long is never going to be perfect, but will have to do. "Call it good," Joe will say. It seemed the right thing to say about the pressure-treated shoes. They weren't ideal, but they would do. My building had fallen into the world.

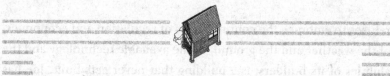

CHAPTER 5

Framing

The corner posts arrived on a snowy January morning, four red plastic flags flapping off the tail of a flatbed. At first I was puzzled. I'd ordered eight six-by-ten timbers—two for each corner of the building—not four. But as the truck backed into the driveway, I realized the mill had simply cut twenty-footers instead of tens, leaving it to me to saw them in half. It made no difference, really, and yet it did. Without meaning to, the mill had made sure I understood these were *trees* they'd sent me from Oregon, not just a pile of lumber.

The yard had sent two men to help unload. A friend of mine also happened to be around, and after taking a few minutes to small-talk and gather ourselves for the task, the four of us slid one of the great timbers off the flatbed and, with a collective groan, hoisted it up onto our shoulders. Moving at an almost ceremonial pace, we walked the massive trunks up the long, snow-crusted incline to the barn, where Joe and I intended to work on our frame indoors until spring.

Whenever more than two people are carrying something as long and heavy as these timbers, it is the tallest person, and not necessarily the strongest, who ends up shouldering the greatest load, and that turned out by a few unlucky inches to be me. One of the guys from the yard estimated that the timbers had to weigh easily a quarter of a ton apiece, and as I felt my share of the load—one quarter of that plus the tallest-guy penalty—grind into the little bone at the top of my shoulder, I started seriously to doubt I could make it all the way to the barn. After awhile all I could think about was how I was going to keep clear of the falling timber when my shoulder—or would it be my knees?—gave out. Struggling to stave off the calamity, I tried to imagine myself as a pallbearer at the funeral of an exceptionally large relative, and rehearsed the shame and embarrassment that would follow were I to drop my end of the load. This did the trick; we made it safely to the barn.

A twenty-foot piece of clear Douglas fir is an impressive thing to behold. By virtue of its girth and length it seems more tree than lumber, though you can easily understand why lumber is what we prefer to call it. Lumber is an abstraction—a euphemism, really. Though these logs had been squared up and dressed at the mill, it was impossible not to be conscious of them as trees—and not to feel at least slightly abashed at what had been done to them on my account. Simply by picking up the phone and placing an order for "eight ten-foot pieces of six-by-ten appearance-grade Doug fir," I'd set in motion a chain of events that was as momentous as it was routine. To fill my order, at least two mature fir trees, green spires as old as the century, had been felled in a forest somewhere in Oregon and then trucked, or floated, to a mill in a town called

McMinnville. This much I knew from the yellow cardboard tag stapled to the endgrain. There they'd been skinned of their bark and, after several passes through a saw and then a planer, transformed into the slabs of salmon-colored lumber that, following a cross-country journey by train, came to lie on the floor of this barn in Connecticut, looking more than a little forlorn.

It's hard not to feel sentimental about such majestic pieces of wood, especially today, when we can appreciate the preciousness of old trees more than we once did. One measure of that preciousness is price. The four timbers in my barn cost more than $600, a figure that manages to seem both exorbitant and—considering what they are, or were—paltry at the same time. Since the corner posts would be a conspicuous element of the interior as well as the exterior of the building, Charlie had specified the highest-grade "clear"—that is, knot-free—fir, wood that is generally found only in the unbranched lower trunks of the oldest trees. It is the fate of precisely such Douglas firs, and the creatures whose habitat depends on them, that loggers and environmentalists have been fighting over in the Pacific Northwest, a fight that has already closed down hundreds of sawmills like the one in McMinnville.

Though I had no paralyzing regrets about taking a couple of these trees, I have to say that what I knew about them, and what I saw before me, did give me pause, heightening the sense of occasion that attended my plans for them. It would be awhile before I felt comfortable putting a saw blade or a chisel to these timbers. You couldn't help feeling responsible for pieces of wood like this, and risking a mistake—*learning* on them, which is after all what I proposed to do—seemed almost unconscionable, a sacrifice of something that had been sacrificed once already.

Had the ton of lumber sitting on the floor of my barn been an equivalent pile of two-by-fours instead, I doubt if any of these thoughts would have crossed my mind. For one thing, ordinary "dimension lumber," as it is called, represents another order of abstraction from the forest. It takes a more strenuous exercise of imagination to see the tree in the two-by-four. For another, the kinds of trees generally used to produce two-by-fours are not the kinds of trees anybody mourns for. In most cases these trees are spindly young specimens harvested from industrial tree farms rather than from forests.

But two-by-fours were not an option for the frame of my building, even though Joe and I would be using plenty of them elsewhere in its construction. Charlie had specified large timbers because our original notion of the building, as a kind of primitive hut carved out of the forest, was unthinkable without them. The archetypal hut consists of four substantial corner posts (actual trees, in some accounts) surmounted by a gable made of timbers only slightly less substantial. A hut's construction should recall the forest from which it springs, and that's more easily done with six-by-ten timbers than sticks of what carpenters call "two-by."*

The primitive hut is a myth, really, a story of the origins of architecture in the state of nature. As the story goes, architecture was given to man by the forest, which taught him how to form a shelter out of four trees, one at each corner, crowned by pairs of branches inclining toward one another like rafters. Like many myths this one is fanciful but also in some deep sense true. For architecture as we know it is unimaginable without the tree. Frank Lloyd Wright, speaking of the very first structures built by man, once wrote that "trees must have awakened his sense of form." It is the tree that gave us the notion of a column and, in the West at least, everything else rests upon that. Even when the Greeks turned from building in wood to stone (after they'd denuded their land of trees), they shaped and arranged their stones in imitation

---

* As anyone who has ever bought lumber quickly discovers, a commercial two-by-four today is actually only 1½″ by 3½″. "Two-by-four" refers to a piece of lumber's rough-sawn dimensions; the sawmill's planer typically removes a half inch, and most commercial lumber dimensions must be adjusted accordingly.

of trees: Greek architecture is based on wooden post-and-beam construction. An architecture utterly ignorant of trees is conceivable, I suppose, but it wouldn't be *our* architecture. Long after the forests are all gone and "wood" has been forgotten, our buildings will still be haunted by trees.

If the idea of a hut dictated the big, treelike timbers, the timbers in turn dictated the building's system of construction. It would be a variation on the traditional post-and-beam, in which the frame of a building is comprised of large and generously spaced vertical posts joined to horizontal beams. Traditionally, these joints were of the type known as mortise and tenon: The end of each beam is chiseled to form a protruding shape called a tenon (from "tongue") that is inserted into a matching notch, or mortise, carved into the post, and then held in place with wooden pegs driven through the two members. Until the 1830s, when carpenters in Chicago invented the modern "balloon frame," in which relatively light pieces of lumber are joined with nails, virtually all buildings built out of wood had post-and-beam frames held together with mortises and tenons.

Traditional post-and-beam joinery requires a specialized set of skills not many carpenters possess anymore, so it seemed unlikely Joe and I would attempt to mortise-and-tenon our frame. Learning how to reliably sink a twelve-penny nail promised to be challenge enough for at least half of this construction crew. Evidently assuming as much, Charlie had proposed a suitably idiot-proof alternative to a traditional joint: his construction drawings called for a steel "joist hanger" at the point where the corner posts joined the four-by-eight beams that would support the floor. A joist hanger is essentially a small steel seat, or sleeve, attached to a vertical plate; the plate gets nailed to the post, and the horizontal beam is dropped into the seat and held in place with common nails. Since this particular joint would be hidden beneath the floor, there was probably no good reason *not* to use a joist hanger.

But Joe didn't see things that way. The afternoon he noticed the joist hanger on the blueprint he evenly but firmly informed me that, no matter what "the architect" had to say about it, no building he was going to work on would use a joist hanger to secure such an important joint. To emphasize the point, he noisily flicked the back of his hand against the offending section of blueprint while he spoke. I suspect that Joe may have been insulted by the drawing, that he'd taken Charlie's spec as an affront to his skill as a carpenter. I tried to explain that it had obviously been *my* competence Charlie had in mind, not his. That might be, Joe said, but the fact remained that steel was not the proper way to join two large wooden members together, and he wasn't about to do it.

Most of the good carpenters I've ever met have a deep devotion to wood and a corollary disdain for steel. Steel might be stronger than wood, but in the mind of many carpenters—especially those carpenters who regard themselves as upholders of a tradition that built a nation out of wood and hardly anything else—steel is still a shade too newfangled to be trusted completely. Steel represents the triumph of industry over craft in construction, and one of the things that draws a person to carpentry today is that it remains one of the few refuges of craft in an industrial economy.

A carpenter like Joe is inclined to think of himself as a guardian of wood's glorious past, if not its sacred honor. Not that Joe is a reactionary on the subject of materials; his time in the body shop has made him more comfortable working with steel than nine out of ten carpenters. But it offended his sense of propriety to join a post to a beam with a joist hanger bought at the hardware store, not when the application of time-tested craft could produce a joint that would not only be more in keeping but would probably last longer too. The fact that nobody would ever see our joint was irrelevant. "That doesn't matter—*we'll* know," Joe said after I made a pitch along these lines for sticking with Charlie's spec. I still regarded the construction drawings as canonical, a habit of mind Joe appeared determined to break. A contest for authority was brewing, and it looked like I was the ground on which it was going to be fought.

What Joe proposed we use in place of Charlie's joist hanger was not, strictly speaking, a true mortise-and-tenon joint. Since the dimensions of the beam (four by eight) were considerably smaller than the post's, we could simply "let" the beam into a four-by-eight notch chiseled into the post, as if the whole beam were a tenon. We would then secure the joint with a bolt, evidently a permissible use of steel. I checked with Charlie, who gently pointed out that this would be an awful lot of work for a detail nobody would ever see. But he had no objection, just so long as we made sure each beam had at least three inches of "bite," or purchase, on its post. So I went out and bought an inexpensive set of wood chisels. Joe had won one—for wood, but also, as I would come to understand, for himself.

≡

Our first day of wood work, Joe showed up with an incongruous pair of tools: a set of fine chisels with ash handles and a fairly beat-up looking chain saw. The chain saw was to cut our posts roughly to length; this would constitute the first cut made in our fir, and as I was afraid he might, Joe insisted that I make it.

I am petrified by chain saws, a phobia I don't regard as irrational or neurotic in the least. It is in fact scientific, being grounded in the laws of probability and the empirical fact of my innate clumsiness and haste in dealing with the physical world. The way I see it, there is only a fixed number of times—unknowable, but certainly not large—that I can expect to use a chain saw before I become the victim of a blood-spurting and possibly life-threatening accident.

Fitting though it may have been to burn up one of those times making the posts for my hut, this didn't mean I was happy about it. Yet there was no way to decline the chain saw Joe held out to me without suffering a loss of face. Though Joe himself is not overbearingly macho, a masculine weather hangs over all construction sites, and it seems to inspirit certain tools in particular—generally the ones that are loudest, most dangerous, and most dramatic in their worldly impact. That puts the chain saw right up there. Joe and I shared no illusions I had any clue what I was doing as a carpenter, but it would have been a mistake to compound my ignorance with a lack of pluck right at the beginning. So, striving manfully for nonchalance, I took the chain saw from Joe, gave its starting cord a yank, and held on tight as the machine leapt menacingly to life.

Cutting the fir timbers proved unexpectedly easy, probably because there were no imperfections in the wood, no knots or bark to frustrate the blade and provoke its willfulness. The snout of the saw moved like a knife through the soft, cheddary wood, its gasoline howl—deafening indoors—the sole evidence of effort or resistance. For the first time, I noticed the sweet, elusive aroma of fresh-cut Doug fir, an oddly familiar perfume that nevertheless took me the longest time to place. But then there it was: roasted peanuts and hot spun sugar, the summery scents of the fairground.

The chain saw gave us four posts each roughly ten feet long; now we had to cut them exactly to length with a circular saw and then lay out the locations of our notches. These particular measurements were not shown on the drawings, however, since they could not be determined without taking certain particularities of the site into account. To arrive at the precise length of the posts, we needed to add the specified height of the walls (shown on the blueprint as 8'1") to the unspecified distance between the top of the rock footings (each of which was slightly different) and the floor. But where exactly *was* the floor? Charlie had left that for us to determine.

Normally the height of a building's floor is determined simply by measuring up from the top of the foundation. But because of the differences among the elevations of our four footings (owing both to the slope of the site and to variations in the size of the boulders), we instead had to fix the floor height at a hypothetical point in space (whatever looked best, basically) and then measure *down* from there to our footings. Every other measurement in the building would be based on the coordinates of this imaginary plane.

Does this sound confusing? It was. "I'm starting to see a pattern here," Joe muttered as we trekked out to the site to make our field measurements. The footings were covered with a foot of snow. "Nothing about this building is normal."

Back in the warmth of the barn, Joe and I each took custody of a post, marking it for length (remembering to subtract 1½″ for the pressure-treated wood shoe it would stand on) and then penciling on its face a 3½″-by-7½″ rectangle where the notch (for our four-by-eight beam) would go. I was eager to start in on my mortise, but Joe had a lesson for the day he wanted to make sure I took to heart: "Measure twice, cut once." Simple as it is, this is one of the carpenter's most important axioms, aimed at averting mistakes and the waste of wood. It proved to be one I had a hard time honoring, however, probably because I was so accustomed to working in a medium in which the reworking of material is not only possible, but desirable. "Undo Typing" is actually one of the commands in my word-processing program, part of a whole raft of options designed expressly to accommodate a writer's haste, sloppiness, or second thoughts. There being no "Undo Sawing" command, the carpenter who makes a mistake is apt to call, in jest, for the "wood stretcher"—a tool that of course doesn't exist. The irreversibility of an action taken in wood is how the carpenter comes by his patience and deliberation, his habit of pausing to mentally walk through all the consequences of any action—to consider fully the implications for, say, the trimming of a doorjamb next month of a cut made in a rafter today. These were alien habits of mind, but ones I'd resolved to learn. So I followed Joe out the door, trudging back into the snow to double-check our measurements.

To trade a chain saw for a chisel is to trade one way of knowing a piece of wood for another. Though the chain saw acquaints you with certain general properties—a wood's hardness and uniformity, its aroma—the chisel discloses much finer information. Something as subtle as the variation in the relative density of two growth rings—the sort of data any machine would overwhelm—the beveled tip of the chisel's steel blade will accurately transmit to its ash handle and through that to your hand.

The chisel enters into the body of the fir tree, and when it is sharp, the material it encounters there feels less like wood than dense flesh. As I tapped on the handle with my ash mallet, the blade sliced easily through its salmon-colored layers, raising a plume of curled shavings I half expected to be moist to the touch. Before a well-honed blade, the substance of a piece of clear Douglas fir yields almost as if it were a slab of tuna. As the chisel slips past the dead outer skin of the timber, the wood brightens and colors, seems more alive.

Once I grew comfortable with the tool, working the fir became thoroughly enjoyable, more pastime than chore. Mortising calls for an appealing mix of attentiveness and mindlessness, keeping part of the mind engaged while setting the rest of it free to wander. Also counting in its favor was the fact that the chisel was a tool that couldn't easily kill me, no matter how badly I mishandled it. Having been put to the same purpose for a few thousand years, the chisel feels supremely well adapted to its task. Its blade has two different faces—one beveled at a forty-five-degree angle, the other straight. The first one wants to dig down deep into the substance of the wood, the second to slip more lightly along its grain, shaving off curls of fir thin enough to let light through them. By rotating the handle of the tool in your hand, you can carefully regulate the amount of wood the blade removes, plunging or shaving depending on how close to the borders of the notch you're working. The challenge is to keep to the outlines you've drawn, being careful not to make the notch any bigger than it absolutely has to be, in order to ensure a snug fit. So every few minutes I'd test my notch by inserting a scrap piece of four-by-eight, which served as understudy for my beam.

After some practice the tool began to feel light and alive in my hands, almost as if it knew what it was supposed to do. Which in some sense it did. Like any good hand tool, but especially one that has been fine-tuned over centuries, a well-made chisel contains in its design a wealth of experience on which the hands of a receptive user can draw. Working properly with such a tool awakens that experience, that particular knowledge of wood; at the same time it helps to preserve it. When the chiseling was going particularly well, it reminded me of what it is like to work with an exceptionally well-trained animal; if I paid close enough attention to what it wanted to do, even let it steer me a bit, the chisel had things to teach me.

After Thoreau cut down the pine trees for the frame of his hut at Walden, he hewed and notched the logs himself, a process—an intimacy, to judge by his account of it—that he believed had somehow righted his relationship to the fallen trees. "Before I had done I was more the friend than the foe of the pine tree," he wrote, even "though I had cut down some of them, having become better acquainted with it." I used to think this was a too-convenient rationalization for Thoreau's having done something that ordinarily he would have deplored. This is, after all, the same Thoreau who once composed an elegy for a pine tree felled by a lumberman ("Why does not the village bell sound a knell?"). Now we are to believe that the care he has taken hewing these pines, the purpose to which he's put them, and the knowledge they have yielded are enough to compensate for the sacrifice. Yet the idea no longer seemed self-serving or crazy, as Thoreau's arguments sometimes do. It was the work that bought this intimate knowledge, the inescapable price of which is the death of a tree. Though it's probably wrong to think that only the handworker, with his traditional tools, gains such an intimate acquaintance with trees; the lumberman working with his screaming chain saw knows trees too, he just knows different things about them. Both, however, come to know the tree better than its more distant admirers.

My own acquaintance with Douglas fir owed as much to the desultory chatter of my chiseling companion (the pace and quiet of the work, which has a lot in common with whittling, is ideal for conversation) as it did to the clinking of my chisel. Going by the number of growth rings, I determined that seventy-five years of tree life were represented in the section I was working; the tree had to be still older than that, however, since the section contained neither its innermost nor outermost ring. As I chiseled my way down to a depth of three inches, slowing as I neared my target, I noticed that the rings were not evenly spaced. The innermost ones were as thick as my finger, and they narrowed as they moved out from the core, until they were so slender as to be barely discernible. According to Joe, this indicated that the tree had probably started life out in the open, allowing it to make rapid growth during its first few years. As the forest grew up around it, however, sunlight became progressively more scarce and the tree's growth slowed accordingly. The pattern suggested my fir tree was probably second-growth, and that it may have been planted on the site of a clear-cut.

I noticed too that each ring was made up of two distinct layers: Rings of reddish-brown, dense-looking wood alternated with ones that were softer and pinkish-yellow in hue. Joe explained that a fir tree puts on two distinct kinds of growth every year. It seems the tree grows very rapidly in the spring, laying down a wide, porous layer of cambium in order to speed the passage of water and nutrients to its flush of new leaves. Growth slows in the summer, and the tree adds a thinner layer of hardwood, the main purpose of which is to strengthen the trunk. Fir is known for laying down a consistently high proportion of strong, dense summerwood, which is what makes it such a good structural timber. As I chiseled, I could feel the difference between spring- and summerwood as a slight change in resistance.

While we worked on our respective notches, Joe and I passed the time talking about the intricacies of post-and-beam construction. The joints we were making were relatively simple ones—no dovetails or, for that matter, true tenons to worry about—but even so, Joe had dozens of tips, big and small, to pass on, most of them having to do with the choice and handling of chisels and the behavior of wood grain; you could see that, behind this process, stood an old and intricate culture of woodwork. But much as I enjoyed making my notches, I was somewhat relieved there weren't many more of them to make. The work proceeded slowly, its progress measured in fractions of inches. You worried constantly about trespassing the borders of your notch, a transgression that couldn't be taken back. When I saw how long it took us to make two mortises in a single post (one to hold the floor beam, another for the header), the idea of erecting an entire building by this method—hewing the timbers, chiseling hundreds of joints far more elaborate than ours, and then raising the frame all by hand—well, all this now seemed about as improbable to me as building a pyramid.

When I grumbled about the cumbersomeness of mortising compared to hammering together a frame of two-by-fours with nails, Joe sprang to the defense of post-and-beam construction. He claimed that timber frames were structurally superior to modern balloon frames (and indeed there are post-and-beam frames from the Middle Ages still standing in Europe) and that they made a more economical use of wood; the additional passes through a saw required to transform a log into two-by-fours wasted far more wood (in the form of sawdust), not to mention energy.

There was a certain poetic economy in post-and-beam framing, in the way it seemed to carry the "treeness" of lumber forward into a building. The vertical posts performed like trunks, exploiting the strength of wood fibers in compression, while the horizontal beams acted very much like limbs, drawing on their strength in tension. And as I realized the first time we fitted a beam into its notch, the two members locked together in a satisfyingly knotlike way; instead of the superficial attachment made by a nail, the beam nested into the body of the post almost as if it were a bough. But, soundness and sentiment aside, it seemed to me that, as much as anything else, it was the very difficulty and mystique of traditional framing that commended it to Joe. Since not everybody could do it, those who could were entitled to a special status.

Up until the second half of the nineteenth century, the joiner, or housewright—to use the two terms by which carpenters were then known—possessed the cultural authority and prestige that architects possess today. They ruled the house-building process from design to completion. And the chief source of the housewright's authority was his expertise in the ways of joining wood timbers, since joinery was easily the most critical and dangerous operation in the making of a building. The status of the carpenter has never fully recovered from the invention of the balloon frame, which replaced posts and beams and mortised joints with slender studs, sills, and joists that just about anybody with a hammer could join with cheap nails. By insisting we mortise our joints, a decision that immediately cast me as his pupil and himself as master, Joe was reclaiming some of the joiner's lost authority for himself. Without challenging Charlie directly, he had removed the making of my building to a time before architects mattered, when the carpenter was sovereign.

≡

The shift from post-and-beam to balloon framing (named for the dubious-seeming lightness of the new structure) marks an important change not only in the history of wood construction, but also in the practice of architecture, the work of building, and even, it seems, in the way that people think about space and place. For between the two types of frame stands a gulf of sensibility as well as technology. This is something my building helped me to at least begin to appreciate, since its frame was a hybrid that acquainted me with both traditions. After Joe and I had raised the front corner posts onto their rock feet and then fitted our floor beams into their notches, we traded our chisels for hammers and nails. The floor, the eighteen-inch "knee wall" at the middle of the building where it stepped down with the ground plane, and the lower sections of its end walls were all to be framed out of conventional two-by-fours and -sixes, in the way most wooden structures have been framed since about 1850 or so.

Now that we were swinging hammers rather than tapping chisels, I felt like I was back on at least semifamiliar ground. But on the first morning of floor framing, I noticed Joe watching me closely as I pounded nails, clearly weighing whether or not to interrupt.

"Can I show you a better way to do that?"

"What—to hammer a nail?" I was incredulous, and then, after he explained what I was doing wrong, crestfallen: it turned out I didn't even know the proper way to swing a hammer. It seems I was holding the side of the hammer with my thumb, a grip that forced my wrist to deliver most of the force needed to drive the nail. Joe reached over and moved my thumb down around the shank of the hammer. Now as I brought the hammer down I felt a slight loss of control but a substantial gain in power, for suddenly the tool had become an extension of my whole arm and not just my hand. Joe never said it, but I'd been holding my hammer as if it were a tennis racket poised for a backhand, a realization that heated my cheeks with embarrassment. Once I'd corrected my grip, I found I could drive a big, ten-penny nail through a piece of two-by with half as many blows as before (this was still twice as many as it took Joe, however), and the business of framing moved smartly along.

It wasn't hard to see why balloon framing had caught on. Where it had taken the two of us to raise and manhandle our posts and beams into position, a process akin to standing a tree trunk on a dime (the dime here being the pin jutting up from the rock through the pressure-treated pad), I was able to frame most of the floor and the entire knee wall by myself in considerably less time than it had taken me to chisel a pair of notches. As soon as I acquired the knack of toe-nailing (angling a nail through the tip of a stud or joist and then into a beam), the work just flew. Only after struggling with six-by-ten posts can you understand how carpenters could ever have thought of two-by-four studs as "sticks"—by comparison, these seemed about as light and easy to handle as toothpicks. Almost without looking, I could pick a two-by-four out of the pile (they were more or less interchangeable), mark it for length, cut it, and toe-nail it into place—all by myself.

Though this wood too was Douglas fir, I was only dimly aware of this fact, and might not have noticed had the yard slipped in a few pieces of spruce or pine. Balloon framing doesn't acquaint you with the particularities of wood in the way post-and-beam framing does, and it's easy to forget these are trees you're working with. It's geometry you worry about—with so many more elements to keep square—rather than the idiosyncrasies of wood. In this sense two-by-four framing is a more abstract kind of work than timber framing, with an industrial rhythm that places a far greater premium on the repetitive task and the interchangeable part. Which is why an amateur like me could frame a knee wall in an afternoon without help from anyone.

What I was discovering in the course of framing my little building, an entire culture had discovered in the middle of the last century. Contemporary accounts of the new technology brim with a kind of giddiness at the rapid feats of construction it had suddenly made possible—houses put up in days, whole towns rising in weeks. "A man and a boy can now attain the same results, with ease, that twenty men could on an old-fashioned frame," wrote one Chicago observer in 1869. There was, too, a lingering skepticism, reflected in the derisiveness of the term "balloon frame," that a structure consisting of nothing more substantial than sticks held together with nails could actually stand up or last. What a revolutionary, and unsettling, notion this must have been; imagine if contractors today were suddenly to start building houses out of cardboard. People thought the new frames looked as flimsy as the baskets they resembled.

Though still a technology based on wood, balloon framing is a product of the machine age: it would never have developed if not for the invention of the steam-powered sawmill (which ensured a ready supply of lumber of consistent dimensions) and manufactured nails. Prior to 1830 or so, nails were hand-forged, making them far too precious to be used in the quantities that a balloon frame required. It was the industrial revolution that, by turning nails into a cheap commodity and trees into lumber, prepared the ground for this radical new way of putting together a building.

But if the machine made the balloon frame possible, it was, more than anything else, the ecology of the Great Plains that made it necessary. In the days before the railroad, timber framing depended on an ample supply of trees too large to be transported any great distance. In most places, building in wood had been essentially a local process of translating the native forest into the various shapes of habitation. But as soon as the American frontier slipped west of Chicago, pioneers found themselves for the first time trying to settle a grassland rather than a forest. It was the development of the balloon frame, with its easily transportable materials, that opened such an ecosystem to settlement. The translation of forest into habitation could now take place on the national rather than local level, with Chicago playing the role of middleman, milling wood from the northern forest and shipping it into the unwooded plains. Chicago, and the balloon frame, had transformed the tree into lumber.

Since a couple of men could assemble one of the new frames without the kind of group effort or specialized skills needed to raise a timber frame, a pioneer family now could build a house just about anywhere they wanted. By comparison, the technology of timber framing—communal and hierarchical by its very nature—had been supremely well adapted to the kind of close-knit religious communities that had settled the forested East. Looked at from this perspective, the new building method added a powerful centrifugal force—and a force for individualism—to the settlement of the American West.

Balloon framing also helped usher in an architectural revolution that would remake both the American house and landscape. Post-and-beam construction had been an inherently conservative building method, not least because of the great number of people it required and the considerable danger involved. In *Common Landscape of America,* the historian John Stilgoe explains that every timber-frame barn builder or house builder "laying out the subassemblies around the floor of his barn understood that his neighbors would devote one day to raising them into position. It was imperative, therefore, that he plan a [structure] immediately familiar to everyone because no one had time to discuss an unfamiliar construction." Since traditional designs were quite dangerous enough, it made good sense for builders to shun novel ones, an imperative that produced an architecture as inflexible, boxy, and rigidly Euclidean as the post-and-beam frame itself. As Stilgoe writes, "raising a strange frame tempted fate."

Not so a balloon frame. This radical new method of cutting and joining trees allowed Americans at mid-century to burst open their post-and-beam boxes and admit the fresh air of architectural originality to their houses. But as much as the new technology, it was the new way of working it made possible—work readily learned and comparatively safe—that changed both the face and the floor plan of the American house. No longer did the house builder need to rely on his neighbors' willingness to risk their necks raising the frame of his home; now he could hire a journeyman or two and swiftly put up any one of the myriad designs, in a bewildering range of styles, being popularized in the new "pattern books," many of which became best-sellers.

Reading about this sea change, just as I was making the switch myself from the rigor of post-and-beam to the relative ease of balloon framing, I began to understand some of the lines of forces that bind the art of architecture to the craft of building. I saw how in a balloon-frame wall I could easily put a window or a door, a room divider or a structural support, just about anywhere I wanted; the rigid syntax of timber framing that insisted on a heavy post every eight or sixteen feet had been repealed, and the specialized skills of the joiner suddenly counted for less than those of the architect. It was the ease and flexibility of this new frame that allowed a thousand architectural flowers to bloom in the second half of the nineteenth century, and eventually made it possible to build the kind of airy and dynamic American space Thoreau had prophesied when he dreamed of a house as "open and manifest as a bird's nest"—a space that could at last accommodate the expansiveness of the American character, being less like a box than, well, a balloon.

=

The first balloon-frame structure in the world was St. Mary's Catholic Church in Chicago, erected by three men in three months in the year 1833. Speed and expedience appear to have been the motive forces. Though fewer than a thousand people lived in Chicago at the time, the infant boomtown was already running short of big trees suitable for timber framing. It did have steam-driven sawmills, however, and logs could be floated down along Lake Michigan from the vast white pine forests of Michigan and Wisconsin. The new building method—which for many years was called "Chicago construction"—allowed the city to be built, if not quite in a day, then in something less than a single year. No one, anywhere, had seen anything quite like it before, an entire city thrown together with the flurry and haste of a campground.

St. Mary's Church was demolished long before anyone had a chance to recognize its historical significance. Which is too bad, but pretty much what you'd expect from an age whose gaze was fixed on the future rather than the past, as well as from a building system that made a virtue not only of speed but of impermanence. Balloon frames are not the stuff of monuments.

But then, it was precisely these qualities that commended the new frame to Americans, who took to it quickly and still rely on it, with some modifications, to build the great majority of their houses. The balloon frame seems to answer to our longings for freedom and mobility, our penchant for starting over whenever a house or a town or a marriage no longer seems to fit. For a people who moves house as often as we do (typically a dozen times in a lifetime) and likes to remodel each house along the way, a balloon frame is the most logical thing to build, since it is not only quick and inexpensive, but easy to modify as well.

J. B. Jackson, the chronicler of America's vernacular landscape, once wrote that "a house is in many ways a microcosm of the landscape; the landscape explains the house." When I first came across this somewhat gnomic observation, we had recently bought our house, and I could not see how Jackson's hypothesis could possibly apply. Like hundreds of thousands of American houses built over the last century, ours was a balloon frame with origins in Chicago: a Sears, Roebuck "ready cut," or kit house built in 1929, it had been selected from among hundreds of floor plans and styles in a catalog, shipped to Cornwall by boxcar, and then nailed together. Had the farmer built his house with fieldstone, I might have understood Jackson's point: certainly this rocky hillside would explain *that* house. But how could this landscape explain a mail-order balloon-frame house?

Jackson recounts a long-running argument in the history of American houses between an Old World tradition of stone building (promoted notably by Thomas Jefferson, who deplored the shoddy wood houses Americans were already in the habit of throwing together) and a more restless New World culture of wood. Beginning during the Renaissance, stone construction replaced timber framing in Europe (the French refer to the housing boom of the six-teenth and seventeenth century as "the victory of stone over wood"), but no such victory ever took place in the colonies. Obvi-ously, the easy availability of wood has a great deal to do with this, but even when trees were scarce, as they were in the Great Plains, we quickly figured out a way to keep building in wood. And in places where brick or stone was an option, as it had been for the farmer, wood continued to hold a powerful appeal. Compared to stone, wood was cheaper, faster, and far easier to adapt to chang-ing circumstances. There was optimism in wood.

Had the farmer who built my house thought he'd be staying here for more than a few years, he might well have used the fieldstone he possessed in such abundance. But to have done so would have implied a happier relationship to the land than he appears to have had, as well as a dimmer view of his prospects in life. The very lightness and impermanence of a balloon frame may have repre-sented to him a form of hope. The farmer didn't mean to put down very deep roots in this rocky soil; why should he, when something better was bound to come along? As soon as it did, he'd shed this place like a chrysalis, no regrets. One did not build a chrysalis out of fieldstone, or even for that matter out of heavy timbers joined together with mortises and tenons. A boxcar full of two-by-fours and a few pounds of nails would do just fine.

≡

I thought about the farmer more than once that spring as we worked on the heavy timber frame of my building. I thought about the speed and ease with which his precut, mail-order frame must have come together; it had taken Joe and me several weeks to get just the front of the structure framed. I also thought about J. B. Jackson's ques-tion, about how the same landscape that "explained" the farmer's mail-order bungalow could also explain a building as different from it as my post-and-beamy hut. But though this might be the same land the farmer had built on, it was no longer quite the same landscape.

It seemed to me that even the posts themselves implied a landscape some distance from the farmer's, one that had welcomed back the same trees (oak and hickory, pine and hemlock) that he would have looked upon as weeds. These massive vertical pairs of exposed six-by-tens—so much bigger than anything a structural engineer would have spec'd for the load, and then doubled up on top of that—called attention to themselves as wood, belonged to a landscape in which trees are prized and people have become self-conscious about preserving them. In part this is because it is a landscape shaped no longer primarily by work but by leisure. The farmer's kit house, with its horizontal clapboards painted white, was the product of a culture that saw virtue in the clear-cutting of forests and was untroubled by a waste of wood we would now consider unconscionable. One ready-cut house catalog of that time made a standing offer to homeowners that would be unthinkable today: "We'll pay you a dollar for every knot you find in our houses." Imagine the amount of wood that had to be wasted in order to produce an entirely knot-free house.

Already the stolidness of these corner posts, with their mortises holding the floor beams in an unshakable embrace, suggested, if not permanence, then at least an intention of staying put on the land that the lightly framed bungalow has always lacked. A timber frame creates (and is created by) a more settled landscape than a balloon frame. Any visitor to the site who knew the first thing about construction made the same crack about my heavy frame: *So how many stories up are you planning to go?* "Overbuilt" was the intended dig; and I suppose that it was. Then they would bang on a six-by-ten with the side of their fist, and when that failed to produce even so much as a wiggle, they'd say: *Well I can see this building's not going anywhere.* Nor the man who built it.

≡

The space for these observations, most of them made sitting on the half-framed floor of my half-framed building, opened up in April, when Joe suffered an injury at work that laid him up for several weeks. He'd been working on a foundation crew, setting and stripping concrete forms, when the bucket of a front-end loader swung around and whacked him square in the back, bruising him badly. In his absence, I had managed to frame the knee wall running across the middle of the building and to notch the rear posts, but there was no way I could now raise them by myself; I couldn't even carry them out here by myself, much less lift them onto their pins and shoes. I'd run up against the fact that timber framing was by its nature communal work, requiring the help of many hands. Finding himself in my predicament, the farmer could have finished his balloon frame alone.

Joe's first day back—he showed up in a corset, moving stiffly—turned out to be one of the project's darkest. Our task had been to raise the rear posts and then run the floor beams from the center knee wall on which they sat to the notches we'd cut for them in the rear posts. It quickly became clear that something was terribly wrong: Neither beam met its intended post at anything even remotely resembling a right angle. One of them missed its mortise by a full two inches—which, in an eight-by-thirteen-foot structure, is to say by a mile. Wordlessly, we both reached for our tapes. We measured and compared the long diagonals, corner to corner, and confirmed that the building had indeed fallen seriously, inexplicably, out of square.

A few steps from the building sits a large, low boulder Joe often repaired to when he needed to study the plans closely or work through a geometry problem, and now he invited me to join him on his rock for a serious head-scratch. "Didn't I say we'd used up too much plumb and level on those front posts?" Joe said, straining to lighten a situation he clearly regarded as grim. He was referring to our relative good fortune in raising the front corner posts and framing the lower portion of the floor. Time and time again the little bubble in the level's window had come to rest dead center in its tube of liquid, an event I learned to await nervously and greet with relief. I'd come to think of the little bubble as a stand-in for people, for our comfortableness in space; level and plumb settled the bubble, stilled its jitteriness, in the same way they settled us, making us feel more at home on the uneven earth.

Joe would often talk about plumb and level and square—trueness—as if they were mysterious properties of the universe, something like luck, or karma, and always in short and unpredictable supply. A surplus one week was liable to lead to a shortfall the next. "We were bound to run out sooner or later, but this, Mike, is grave." I knew, at least in an intellectual way, that squareness was an important desideratum in a building, but part of me still wasn't sure why it was *such* a big deal. If the problem wasn't evident to the eye, then how much could a few degrees off ninety really matter? Why should builders make such a fetish of right angles—of something as old-fashioned as "rectitude"? I mentioned to Joe there were architects around, called deconstructivists, who maintained that Euclidean geometry was obsolete. They designed spaces that were deliberately out of plumb, square, and sometimes even level, spaces that set out purposefully to confound the level's little bubble, and in turn our conventional notions of comfort. "Straight," "level," "plumb," "true": in the postmodern lexicon, these terms are . . . well, square. So why couldn't our building afford an acute angle or two? Joe cocked one eye and looked at me darkly, an expression that made plain he regarded my hopeful stab at non-Euclidean geometry as an instance not of apostasy but madness.

"Mike, you don't even want to know all the problems that a building this far out of square is going to have. Trust me—it is your worst nightmare."

Sitting there on Joe's rock, pondering the mystery, we were able to come up with two plausible explanations for what had happened. Both were equally depressing, though in very different ways. Either it was human error in the placement of one of the front posts on its rock, or an act of God involving movement of the rear footings. Earlier that spring we had observed a tremendous amount of groundwater coming through the site (something a fêng shui doctor would doubtless have foreseen). The ground was saturated in March, and as the earth around our footings thawed, we could actually hear gurgling sounds deep underfoot, as if a stream were passing directly beneath us. Could the force of the groundwater actually have moved a four-foot concrete pier? Joe claimed it was possible.

I personally found it difficult to accept that an act of God, or nature, was responsible for throwing our building out of square. To endorse this view might exonerate our workmanship, but it raised too many uncomfortable questions about foundations—about the dependability of the frost line and the very possibility of ever safely grounding a building. I was more inclined to think human error was the cause—what Joe called an "act of idiocy," as opposed to an act of God—and I worked out a scenario in which a seemingly trivial bit of carelessness in the placement of one of our little pressure-treated post "shoes" could have caused the calamity without our realizing it. I may have been more right than I knew when I said they were the building's Achilles' heel.

Thinking back on it, I did have this vagueish memory involving the shoe under the outside northwest post—about how it might have sat a little funny when we put it down on the rock that final time, as if it had been turned around or flipped over. If so, then the entire northwest corner of the building was twisted slightly in space, which would be enough to account for the discrepancies we'd found in the rear posts.

The error, this simple, stupid, unconscious, un-undoable error, haunts my building even now. For although Joe and I were able with great difficulty to make some adjustments in the placement of the rear posts (by shifting where they fell on their rocks, and rotating one of the rocks on its pier), we were never able to entirely rectify the problem—and therefore, the building, which we estimate to be approximately two degrees out of square. As a result, the front wall of my building is slightly more than an inch wider than the back.

Not that it's anything anyone's ever going to notice. At the casual, phenomenological level of everyday life, a building a couple degrees out of square is no big deal. Unfortunately for me, that is not the level at which I elected to have this experience. And at the considerably less forgiving level of experience where rafters have to get cut and desktops scribed, it has been exactly what Joe promised it would be: a nightmare. The whole of the rest of the project has been a seminar in the consummate beauty, if not the transcendental necessity, of square, something I now look back upon wistfully as a lapsed state of architectural grace. Cast out of square, I've learned more than I care to know about the stern and unforgiving syntax of framing, in which any departure from geometrical rectitude ramifies through the world of the structure without end, a dilating, unstoppable stain, an ineradicable corruption. Every step taken since the flip of that shoe has been dogged by those two degrees: Every pair of rafters has had to be cut to a slightly different length; every floorboard and windowsill, every piece of trim and flashing, has an eighty-eight-degree angle somewhere in it, the indelible watermark of our stupidity. Even now, years later, consequences rear up in reminder. When I want to add another shelf to hold my books, I'm quickly reminded that no straightforward rectangle will do. No, I must lay out and cut, then sand and finish and dismayingly behold, the subtlest of trapezoids, a precise off-key echo of the building as a whole. It has been a most exquisite form of penance.

≡

But if framing had given the building its darkest day, cleaving it once and for all from geometrical perfection, it also gave us a few of its brightest: banner days of swift progress and high spirits in which the building literally rose up and took shape before our eyes, almost as if in time-lapse. By Memorial Day, all eight corner posts were standing, along with the upper and lower beams connecting them front to back, and the entire subfloor had been nailed down—faintly trapezoidal, it's true, but I'm proud to say dead-on, bubble-stillingly level.

The weather that June was particularly fine, and many hands mustered. Especially on the Saturday that spring turned into summer, when Judith and I threw a barbecue for a dozen or so friends that turned the following morning into an impromptu frame-raising party. Those who weren't at ease swinging hammers stood around the site and gabbed, watching the kids and shooting video of the doings above, while a handful of us climbed up into the frame, under a fine canopy of new leaves, and nailed into place the sweet-smelling planks of freshly cut fir passed up from below. Isaac was two months shy of his first birthday, and I have a snapshot Judith took of the two of us on the site that splendid afternoon. I'm ferrying lumber to the framers from a stockpile in the barn, all the while carrying Isaac in a pack on my back; OSHA would not have approved. Isaac's got nothing but a diaper on, and his tiny pink hand is reaching up to steady the two-by-six balanced on my shoulder.

Charlie was also on hand, and Joe was due but running more than his usual couple of hours behind schedule. (The man might be a master of space, but time is another matter altogether.) On this occasion, though, there may have been extenuating circumstances. For this was to be Joe and Charlie's first face-to-face, a prospect neither of them relished.

Before Joe arrived we worked on the foot-wide Doug fir plank that Charlie had spec'd to span the tops of the corners posts and tie all four walls together. Like a great many components of the building's frame, this one performed several distinct functions at once, some structural, others formal or ornamental. Structurally, the plank functions as the top plate of the walls, stiffening the frame all around while providing a header for the windows and a seat for the rafters. Inside, the same member serves as the topmost bookshelf, articulating the depth and height of the thick walls that run the length of the building's long sides. Then, at either end of the building, three inches of the plate extend through the wall, jutting out to form a ledge, or lip, on the front and rear elevations, which crowns the corner posts much like a slender cornice. This is its formal role: by establishing a strong, crisp line across the face of the building and defining the base of the pediment, the plank (in combination with the visor in front) gives all the columns something to "die into," thereby resolving the problem of how to terminate the two inner posts. Charlie prepared an axonometric drawing to show us how the cornice plate was supposed to work:

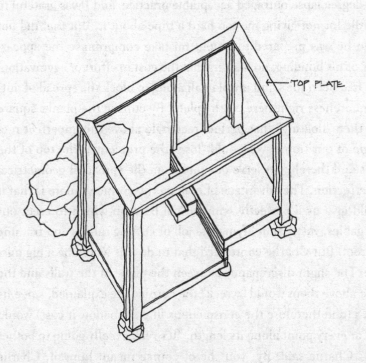

The cornice is exactly the sort of elegantly economical detail I might never have appreciated had I not worked on it directly. With the cornice Charlie had pushed the possibilities of "articulated" structure as far as he could, enlisting the building's frame in the structure of its thick walls and then bringing that interior element out into the design of the exterior elevation. (Though I hasten to add that this is strictly an architect's concept of economy: Since the detail was so important, Charlie had insisted we build the cornice using the clearest, and very dearest, grade of fir.)

As we waited for Joe to show up, Charlie climbed up into the frame to help me lay out our four planks, a procedure that very quickly brought him up to speed on the whole squareness issue. He was doing his best to be nonchalant about it too, though I could see that so messy and steep a declension from the structure he had drawn clearly disturbed him. From an architect's point of view, our two-degree lapse outraged acceptable practice, and I was grateful to Charlie for not giving me too hard a time about it. But that did not mean he was prepared to let our mistake compromise the appearance of his building, no matter what the cost in effort or aggravation.

It had been Joe's and my plan all along to block the spread of out-of-squareness right here, at the plate. By cutting the planks square and then "floating" that perfect rectangle above the imperfect rectangle of our frame, we would "lose" the problem at the top of the walls and thereby preserve our roof from the spread of geometrical imperfection. The advantage of making the cornice square is that it would give us a perfectly symmetrical base on which to erect our two gables, vastly simplifying the job of cutting rafters and framing the roof. But Charlie contended that to do this would be a big mistake. The slight discrepancy between the plane of the walls and the plate above them would "wreck" the cornice, he explained, since its depth (and therefore the conspicuous line of shadow it cast) would vary at every point along its length. "It's really, *really* going to bother you," Charlie said. By "you" he of course meant himself; Charlie had become fully as proprietary about the building as Joe and I were. I couldn't decide whether it was a good or a bad thing that Joe wasn't around to argue the point with him.

Charlie wanted us to cut the plates to match the imperfect frame, thereby pushing the squareness problem up into the rafters, where it would be more or less out of view. "I'm not saying it won't be a headache," he acknowledged. "You're going to be cutting every pair of rafters individually, each to a slightly different length. But then—I promise—it'll be over, the problem won't go any further than that." How could it? The *building* didn't go any further than that. But it seemed to me that if Charlie felt this strongly about the cornice detail, it was probably wise to go along.

Charlie and I were already nailing down the untrued cornice planks when Joe finally appeared, trudging up the hill to the site elaborately festooned with power tools and extension cords. He had on red, white, and blue suspenders, circa 1969, and a pair of trousers, which immediately set him apart from the weekend carpenters on hand in our shorts. Charlie and I came down off our ladders for the introductions, and the two of them shook hands— carefully. Charlie launched an initial foray into geniality, complimenting Joe on his craftsmanship, but when the gesture wasn't reciprocated, he promptly chomped a few nails between his teeth, climbed back up his ladder, and returned to the plank he'd been spiking. It was not a comfortable moment, and the news I had for Joe about the planks did not promise to improve it. I remember thinking: *Men!*

When I told Joe how we'd decided to handle the cornice plate, he gave a shrug of what I knew to be feigned indifference: the two of us had been going back and forth about whether or not to square these planks for weeks as we framed up the side walls, so I knew he had strong feelings on the subject. "Mike, it's your building," he now mumbled, by which I was meant to understand, *and not Charlie's.* Then he looked up at the architect, swinging his hammer on top of the wall, and invited him to come back and help out again the following weekend, and all the weekends after that, when we'd *still* be custom-cutting rafters. "Because framing this roof is shaping up as a *real* good time!"

Charlie laughed off the barb and, to my enormous relief, set to work mollifying Joe. You could see the years of experience smoothing the feathers of all those prickly contractors Charlie's drawings and directives and punch lists had propelled into orbit. By turns self-deprecating, appreciative, and deferential, Charlie managed within moments to assure Joe he had no intention of challenging his authority on the job site. And by the end of the afternoon, Joe was abundantly himself again, handing out orders to everybody, holding forth on politics (the mendacity of government, the people's Second Amendment right to bear arms), and offering design suggestions that Charlie accepted with exceptional good grace.

Later that afternoon, after the architect had headed back to Cambridge, Joe told me Charlie was not at all what he'd expected. "He's almost a regular guy," Joe said. He seemed genuinely astonished.

≡

The episode of the cornice did not mark the cessation of hostilities between Joe and Charlie, however. A certain tenseness would color all their dealings right to the end, now and again flaring in such a way as to strand me uncomfortably in between. I soon learned never to cite Charlie or his plans as a final authority on any question, and always to claim any suggestion from the architect as my own. But Joe wasn't the only party intent on jealously guarding his prerogatives. If I had occasion to mention to Charlie that Joe and I planned to decide on our own some detail left unclear on the blueprint (the framing of a window, say, or the precise depth of the bookshelf walls), he'd urge us to hold off and then, within hours, fax me a drawing in which Joe would then proceed to poke holes.

What was going on here? The project represented only the tiniest of commissions for Charlie, and for Joe it was only fill-in work, a short-term weekend job. Yet both were behaving as if something much more important were at stake.

Of the two, Joe's investment in the project was somewhat easier to fathom. For one or two days every week, and provided Charlie stayed in Cambridge, Joe enjoyed a measure of freedom and authority he had probably never known on the job. He was the foreman, the brains of the operation, the mentor—and I met the payroll. Plus he got to give an architect a hard time whenever he felt like it, evening an ancient score on behalf of carpenters everywhere. You don't find too many deals quite this sweet.

On most construction sites today, the battle between architects and contractors is largely past, if not forgotten. Carpenters may still grumble, but only among themselves, and rarely to any effect; everyone understands that, really, the game is over, and it was the architects who won. Carpenters might still possess a greater degree of autonomy than other workers in an industrial economy, but their authority is a ghost of what it was. In many respects my job was a throwback. The complexity of the design combined with my own inexperience put Joe in a position of unusual power, and never more so than during the work of framing. His role was much like that of the housewright of old, who was typically the only "expert" in a house-raising, directing a crew of amateurs nearly as rank as I. To watch Joe up in the frame, moving from beam to beam with a simian agility, barking orders, galvanizing a crew of incompetents in a procedure as intricate as the raising of a roof, was to watch a carpenter in his glory—and to have some idea what the glory days of the trade must have been like.

But if the carpenter lost out in the war with architects, then what exactly had the architects won? This question helped me to at least begin to understand what my building meant to Charlie. Certainly an architect wields far greater authority than a carpenter. Yet unless he happens to be one of a small handful of stars, his authority too is heavily checked and compromised—by the whims of clients, the imperatives of the marketplace, the dominion of the building code, the rule of popular taste. To the extent that money is a measure of power, the fact that architects are frequently the poorest paid of all the trades on a construction site indicates that the victory of the profession might be, if not hollow, then certainly less resounding than the popular image of the autonomous architect-artist would suggest. The architect as romantic hero has been a powerful stereotype for most of this century, but I think most architects today understand it as the myth that it is. To an architect of Charlie's generation, Ayn Rand's Howard Roark, a character whose name you can't pronounce without hearing the word "heroic," is a figure of fun.

And yet that figure—solitary and utterly uncompromising as he bends the world to his visionary purposes—is perhaps more alluring to architects than they can safely let on. For who *wouldn't* want the career of the romantic hero-artist, breaking free of the shackles of budget and client and marketplace? It's one thing to know better, to understand that architecture is in fact—as it should be—an impure and collaborative art form, but it's quite another to give up completely such a seductive image—the very image, in all likelihood, that attracted you to architecture in the first place.

Maybe I shouldn't speak for Charlie, but I imagine that the "writing house" commission stirred whatever romantic inclinations he might still harbor. In a practice demanding more than its share of prose, the writing house offered at least the chance for poetry. The client had pretty much given the architect his head, the program had an unusual simplicity to it, and there were so few of the usual earthbound considerations to worry about: no plumbing, no insulation, and not a whole lot of building code. In a more conventional project, a detail as elegant as a cornice that passes through the building's skin would almost certainly have been sacrificed to the prosaic need for thickly insulated walls. Freed from such mundane considerations, Charlie could articulate whatever of the building's structure he wanted to, and in doing so design an uncommonly pure work of architecture, his own personal interpretation of the primitive hut.

From one perspective Charlie and Joe would appear to have much in common here—not in their interests, which were bound to clash, but in their motives and aspirations. Both had found in the writing house a degree of freedom and authority, of power really, such as their workaday lives rarely afforded. On this tiny stage, both could play the hero. (And at my expense, in every sense of the word.) The only problem was, the heroism of one had to contend with the heroism of the other.

Leaving aside these conflicts, as well as my own junior status, the project offered all three of us many of the same satisfactions. There was a measure of poetry in the work itself, if only in the sense that we were doing it freely and for ourselves, with no thought to the marketplace. And this was real work too, something more than mere labor—time put in for pay. It was work with a clear beginning, middle, and end. At the end we would have something to show for it, would have added something to the stock of reality—to what Hannah Arendt once called the "huge arsenal of the given." In *The Human Condition* Arendt writes of the privileged position of *homo faber,* man the maker of things, whom the Greeks believed stood not only above the laborer, but above even the man of action and the man of thought, or words. The laborer produces nothing lasting he can call his own, and both the man of action and the man of thought are ultimately dependent on other people, without whose regard and remembrance their deeds and creations do not matter or endure. "*Homo faber* is indeed a lord and master," she writes, "not only because he . . . has set himself up as the master of all nature but because he is master of himself and his doings." At one time or another I think all three of us felt a glimmer of that mastery; we just had to take turns.

≡

The culmination of timber framing arrives with the raising of the ridge pole, a moment of high drama that Joe approached as one of his biggest scenes. For weeks now, I'd been asking him how we were going to do it—should I be lining up some sort of crane for the

day?—and for weeks Joe'd been telling me not to worry, that he'd figure out something when the time came. But it was definitely on his
mind. During breaks, I'd follow his gaze as it slowly traveled up from
the wall plate to the overhanging trees only to suddenly plunge
again; I guessed he was testing out scenarios (a block and tackle?
Maybe a pulley?), running calculations on what it would take to lift
a four-by-ten ridge beam sixteen feet overhead. What I wanted to
know was, did the rafters come first, or the ridge beam? It looked like
a classic chicken-and-egg problem to me: Without a ridge beam,
what's to hold the rafters in place? And without rafters to hold the
ridge beam up, it seemed like you'd need to temporarily levitate the
thing. To me, it looked like another pyramid deal: inconceivable
without a really big rig and a *lot* of guys. But if Joe was nervous about
it—and I think he was, a little—he did a good job of hiding it, all the
while building suspense in his rapt audience of one.

On the July Saturday we proposed to raise the roof beam, Joe
showed up before eight, brimming with determination and confidence. We began indoors, framing the two end gables. Joe worked
his pencil, calculating lengths and angles, then called these out to
me; I manned the table saw. Before a single nail was driven, we laid
the whole assembly out on the floor. Each gable was an isosceles
right triangle consisting of a four-by-six rafter on each of two sides,
a cross beam of the same dimension (known as a collar tie) along
the base, and a four-by-four king post down the middle.

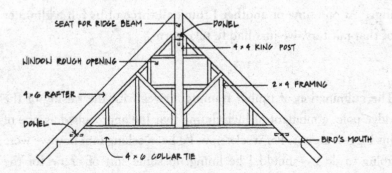

At the apex of this triangle we left a 3½"-by-9" gap between the two rafters and above the post: This was the slot in which the four-by-ten ridge pole would ultimately sit. The one-word answer to my chicken-and-egg riddle was "plywood": we nailed a triangle of half-inch ply to the back of these members to keep them fixed in place until the ridge pole was up. Joe at last unveiled his plan: We would raise the gables into place at either end of the building and then drop the ridge pole into their two pockets. Only after that would we nail the rest of the rafters into place. It sounded to me as though you still wanted the crane (the gable ends themselves weighed several hundred pounds a piece), but Joe said all we would need was one more pair of hands, no particular skill required. So I arranged for an exceptionally tall friend named Don to come by later that afternoon.

The gable ends themselves presented a complicated bit of framing. Owing to our squareness problem, the rear gable had to be an inch and a half narrower than the front, which meant we had to cut the bird's mouth, or notch, on each of the two pairs of rafters at a slightly different spot in order to maintain the same pitch from one end of our roof to the other. (The precise location of these cuts was determined by a complicated formula that Joe worked out to his satisfaction on a scrap of plywood but failed to make intelligible to me.) Then we doweled the joints where the rafters and king post each met the cross beam, pounding a cylinder of hardwood through holes drilled into each member; the dowels would help prevent the roof from splaying outward under the weight of snow.

Typical of this building's design, the gable mixed traditional and modern stud-framing techniques. For nested within the beefy timbers forming the three sides of the gable was a second pattern of lighter members, two-by-fours that held the wall rigid and framed the pair of boxes that would eventually hold the little windows under the peak. Once we had mitered and nailed together these pieces, the gable assemblies were ready to be raised. Somehow.

We carried the first gable out to the site and laid it down on the subfloor. Joe spent a long time just staring up at the top of the wall and then down at the gable. The assembly was far too heavy to be simply passed up onto the wall plate without a small army of helpers top and bottom. Joe now carefully arranged a pair of ladders and set a two-by-ten plank across the tops of the walls; I could see that the trees overhead no longer figured in his calculations.

"Okay, Mike, here's the plan. First we turn the gable upside down and backwards. Then, together, we lift the thing just high enough so that this rafter tail here hits *that* spot there on the plate. You're going to have to balance everything right on that point just long enough for me to climb up onto the top of the wall. Then we pivot the whole assembly this way until the other rafter tail hits that point over there, and then slide the two-by-ten under the peak to hold it up. Follow me? Then I steady the assembly while you get up on the second ladder there, and together we flip the thing around, shimmy it into place, and then get under and lift it to vertical." No, it made no sense to me either, none whatsoever. I told Joe following his plan was like trying to learn origami over the radio. He wasn't smiling, and I realized then that what we were about to attempt was not without danger. I said to Joe that maybe it would be better if he just told me what to do one step at a time.

And so I followed his instructions, moving first this way and then that, hoisting, holding, pivoting, and then climbing on cue, an obedient pyramid ant, not even aspiring to grasp the big picture, and trusting utterly in my carpenter-turned-choreographer. And then, astoundingly, there we were, each of us holding one side of a three-hundred-pound assembly that we'd managed somehow to raise high into the trees without a crane. I wanted to cheer, except that I was still holding my breath as I waited for Joe to brace the gable. So instead I thought about this newspaper article I'd read recently that said that men are more adept than women at mentally rotating an object in space, a skill I'd never had occasion to think about, much less appreciate, before. Women supposedly have the edge in verbal agility, which seemed much the better deal. Not today. Here it was, right in front of me, a full-dress display of the male genius.

We braced the gable with a pair of two-by-fours, and broke for lunch.

≡

It was imperative we get the ridge pole up before the day was out; without it, an errant gust was liable to make a sail of our gable assembly, bring the whole thing crashing down. After lunch we raised the second gable without incident and took a field measurement to determine the precise length of the ridge pole: 13′ 9¼″. This turned out to be a couple of inches less than the dimension shown on Charlie's plan, but then at this point the building had its own reality, of which our mistakes formed a necessary part.

Don, the six-and-a-half-foot friend I'd recruited for the event, arrived as Joe and I were preparing to mark and cut the gorgeous length of knot-free fir we'd selected for the building's spine. This timber too had come from Oregon, according to the stencil on its flank. My tentativeness handling such a piece of wood had vanished; I felt well acquainted with fir—if not quite friend, not foe either. I took up the circular saw, found my mark, and worked the blade through the familiar wood flesh, breathing in its sweet fairground scent. Don, who has some of the lassitude you often find in very lanky people, seemed slightly horrified at just how big the beam was.

"*This* is what you call a ridge pole? I was picturing something a bit more bamboolike."

"We call it a ridge pole to make it feel lighter," Joe said. "But it's really a big tree with the bark taken off and a few corners added."

As the three of us shouldered the ridge pole from the barn out to the site, I thought back to the arrival of the corner posts on a winter morning six months before. Everything about this day seemed infinitely superior: the soft July air, the auspiciousness of the occasion, and the convenient fact that, this time around, mine was not the tallest shoulder underneath this massive tree. Don complained all the way out to the site.

Joe had stationed himself midway between Don and me, but as we neared the site he slipped out from under the beam (since he's five-four, our burden scarcely changed) and trotted out ahead, climbing up into the frame to receive the ridge pole from us. Don, straining, pressed his end up over his head barbell-style while Joe guided it to a spot on the wall plate; then I did the same with my end. Working now nine feet off the ground, we drilled holes at each end of the ridge beam at the spot where it would set down onto the dowels we'd already mounted on the supporting king posts in our gable assemblies. Joe then directed the two of us in a new choreography of lumber that had Don and I manning opposite gables while he flew back and forth across the frame, helping us each in turn to hoist and then align our beam ends over their intended dowels. Don's end went down first, sinking comfortably into its wooden pocket; I watched his tensed expression suddenly bloom into relief, mixed with a satisfaction he hadn't been prepared for. My end took some manhandling, first to align the hole above the dowel, and then to force the beam all the way down into its slot, where it didn't seem to want to go.

"Time for some physical violence," Joe advised, and he handed his big framing hammer up to me. Now I pounded mightily on the top of the ridge beam—holding the hammer correctly, I might add—and inch by inch it creaked its way down onto the dowel, the tight-binding wood screeching furiously under the blows, until at last the beam came to rest on its king post, snug and immovable. That was it: the ridge pole set, our frame was topped out.

I asked Joe to hand me his big carpenter's level; along with the tool he gave me a look that said, You're really asking for it, aren't you? There was nothing we could do, after all, if we discovered that our ridge beam was not true. I laid the level along the spine of the building as close to its midpoint as I could reach. From where he stood Joe had the better view into the level's little window, and I read the excellent news in his face. "It doesn't get any better," Joe said, reaching out his hand for a slap. None of us wanted to come down from the frame, so we stood up there in the trees for a long time, beaming dumbly at one another, weary and relieved, savoring the sweetness of the moment.

≡

In Colonial days the topping out of a frame was traditionally followed by a ceremony, and though the particulars varied from place to place and over time, certain elements turn up in most accounts. According to historian John Stilgoe, as soon as the ridge beam was set into place, the weary carpenters would begin pounding on the frame, "calling for wood." Answering the call, the master builder would go off into the woods to cut down a young conifer and carry it back to the assembled helpers. As the tree sacrifice suggests, the flavor of these events was strongly pagan, even in Puritan America, though there was an effort in many places to work in a few Christian elements, such as the Lord's Prayer. Often there would be some kind of test of divination: in one, the master builder would drive an iron spike into an oak beam, and if the wood didn't split or bleed (being oak, it hardly ever did), the long life of both frame and owner was assured. Toasts and prayers followed, and then a bottle would be broken over the frame in a kind of christening. Many frames were actually given names; "the Flower of the Plain" was one I especially liked. After a toast to the workers and their creation, writes Stilgoe, "The harmony of builders, frame, and nature was assured, and the men raised the decorated conifer to the highest beam in the structure and temporarily fixed it. Thereafter the frame had the life of a living tree."

"Keep all lightning and storms distant from this house," went one common prayer, "keep it green and blossoming for all posterity."

The only part of the traditional topping-out ceremony that has come down to us more or less intact is the nailing of the evergreen to the topmost beam. Even on a balloon-frame split-level in the suburbs, you'll often see an evergreen bough tacked to the gable or ridge board before the vinyl siding goes on. I've seen steelworkers raising whole spruce trees to the top of a skyscraper frame high above midtown Manhattan. Perhaps it's nothing more than superstition, men in a dangerous line of work playing it safe. Or maybe there's some residual power left in the old pagan ritual.

I've read many explanations for the evergreen hanging, and all of them are spiritual in one degree or another. The conifer is thought to imbue the frame with the tree spirit, or it's meant to sanctify the home, or to appease the gods for the taking of the trees that went into the frame. These interpretations sound reasonable enough, and yet they don't account for the fact that someone as unsuperstitious and spiritually backward as me felt compelled to go out into the woods in search of an evergreen after we'd raised the ridge pole. Joe probably would have done it if I hadn't, but it was my building, and there was something viscerally appealing about the whole idea, the way it promised to lend a certain symmetry to the whole framing experience, tree to timber to tree, bringing it full circle. But now that I've performed the ritual, I'm inclined to think there may be more to it than that. Like many rituals involving a sacrifice, there's a kind of emotional wrench in the middle of this one. The hanging of the conifer manages all at once to celebrate a joyful rite—the achievement of the frame and the inauguration of a new dwelling—and to force a recognition that there is something slightly shameful in the very same deed.

People have traditionally turned to ritual to help them frame and acknowledge and ultimately even find joy in just such a paradox of being human—in the fact that so much of what we desire for our happiness and need for our survival comes at a heavy cost. We kill to eat, we cut down trees to build our homes, we exploit other people and the earth. Sacrifice—of nature, of the interests of others, even of our earlier selves—appears to be an inescapable part of our condition, the unavoidable price of all our achievements. A successful ritual is one that addresses both aspects of our predicament, recalling us to the shamefulness of our deeds at the same time it celebrates what the poet Frederick Turner calls "the beauty we have paid for with our shame." Without the double awareness pricked by such rituals, people are liable to find themselves either plundering the earth without restraint or descending into self-loathing and misanthropy. Perhaps it's not surprising that most of us today bring one of those attitudes or the other to our conduct in nature. For who can hold in his head at the same time a feeling of shame at the cutting down of a great oak, and a sense of pride at the achievement of a good building? It doesn't seem possible.

And yet right here may lie the deeper purpose of the topping-out ceremony: to cultivate that impossible dual vision, to help foster what amounts to a tragic sense of what we do in nature. This is something that I suspect the people who used to christen frames understood better than we do. To build, their rituals imply, is in some way to alienate ourselves from the natural order, for good and bad. The cutting down of trees was an important part of it. But even before that came the need for a shelter in the first place—something that Adam had no need for in paradise. Like the clothes Adam and Eve were driven by shame to put on, the house is an indelible mark of our humanity, of our difference from both the animals and the angels. It is a mark of our weakness and power both, for along with the fallibility implied in the need to build a shelter, there is at the same time the audacity of it all—reaching up into the sky, altering the face of the land. After Babel, building risked giving offense to God, for it was a usurpation of His creative powers, an act of hubris. That, but this too: *Look at what our hands have made!*

I don't think it is an accident that the ceremonies came at the point they did in the building process, since it is the setting of the ridge beam that completes the shape of this symbol of our humanity: the gable crowning the square, the very idea of *house* written out in big timbers for all the world to see. The topping-out rituals performed by the early builders, with their peculiar mix of solemnity and celebration, must have offered them a way to reconcile the simultaneous shame and nobility of this great and dangerous accomplishment.

I'm more than a little embarrassed to utter any such words in connection with my own endeavor, so distant from my world do they sound. But along with the remnants of the old rituals, might there also be at least some residue of the old emotions? I remember, on that January morning when I took delivery of my fir timbers, how the sight of those fallen, forlorn timbers on the floor of my barn had unnerved me—"abashed" was the word I'd used. In the battle between the loggers and the northern spotted owl, I'd always counted myself firmly on the side of the owls. But now that I wanted to build, here I was, quite prepared to sacrifice not only a couple of venerable fir trees in Oregon, but a political conviction as well. I was also prepared to make a permanent mark on the land.

So maybe it was shame as much as exultation that brought me down off the frame that early summer evening, sent me out into the woods in quest of an evergreen to kill. Joe had forgotten which you were supposed to use, pine or hemlock or spruce. I decided any conifer would do. It was spruce I came upon first, and after I cut the little tree down and turned to start back to the site, holding the doomed sapling before me like a flag, I saw something I hadn't really seen before: the shape of my building in the landscape. The simple, classical arrangement of posts and beams, their unweathered grain glowing in the last of the day's light, stood in sharp relief against the general leafiness, like some sort of geometrical proof, chalked on a blackboard of forest. I stopped for a moment to admire it, and I filled with pride. The proof, of course, was of us: of the powers—of mind, of body, of civilization—that could achieve such a transubstantiation of trees. *Look at this thing we've made!* And yet nothing happens without the gift of the firs, those green spires sinking slowly to earth in an Oregon forest, and it was this that the spruce recalled me to. Joe had left a ladder leaning against the front gable. I climbed back up into the canopy of leaves, the sapling tucked under my arm, and when I got to the top I drove a nail through its slender trunk and fixed it to the ridge beam, thinking: *Trees!*

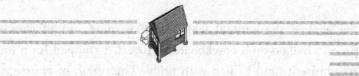

CHAPTER 6

The Roof

Building a roof is by its very nature conducive to speculation, if only because one spends so much of the day so high up in the trees, taking in the big picture. In fact, the process of shingling a roof in wood is the sort of repetitive operation that actually benefits from a certain distractedness on the part of the shingler. Focus too closely on the work at hand and your shingles are apt to fall into a rigid, mechanical pattern, when it's a more organic regularity, something just this side of casual, that you're looking for. This I managed to achieve (shingling obviously played to my strength, such as it is), and perhaps the following reflections on roofs, and other elevated matters, deserve part of the credit.

To think about roofs is to think about architecture at its most fundamental. From the beginning, "the roof" has been architecture's great synecdoche; to have "a roof over one's head" has been to have a home. The climax of every primitive hut narrative I've read arrives with the invention of the roof, the big moment when the tree limbs are angled against one another to form a gable, and then covered with thatch or mud to shut out the rain and the heat of the sun. If the first purpose of architecture is to offer a shelter against the elements, it then stands to reason that the roof is in some sense its primary creation. It's the place where the dreams of architecture meet the facts of nature.

The roof also seems to be the place where, in this century, architecture and nature parted company, where the ancient idea that there are rules for the art of building that are given with the world— an idea first expressed by Vitruvius, and embodied in the myth of the primitive hut—went, well, out the window. At first the notorious leaking roofs of contemporary architecture seemed too cheap and obvious a metaphor for this development. But my time up in the rafters roofing and dwelling on roofs eventually got me to thinking that the leaky roof, taken seriously, might in fact have something to tell us about the architecture of our time.

But before I could think too hard about roofs as metaphor, I needed to learn something about them as structure, if I hoped to get mine framed and shingled and weather-tight that summer before the cold weather returned. Frank Lloyd Wright, who made much of roofs in his work (and who designed more than his share of leaky ones), wrote in his account of mankind's earliest builders that "The lid was troublesome to him then and has always been so to subsequent builders." Roofs have always been the focus of a considerable amount of technological effort, since, as Wright noted, "more pains had to be taken with these spans than with anything else about the building." We tend to forget that, for much of its history, architecture stood at the leading edge of technology, not unlike semiconductors or gene splicing today. The architect saw himself less as an artist than a scientist or engineer, as he pushed to span ever-bigger spaces, to build higher and higher, and to realize such marvels of engineering as towers and domes. Historically, the roof has been the place where architecture confronted the challenge not only of the elements, but of nature's laws.*

Perhaps this accounts for a certain anxiety that seems to hover over a roof, even one as seemingly straightforward as mine. It had never occurred to either Joe or me that our simple forty-five-degree gable roof was in any way pushing the technological envelope, but, unbeknownst to us, Charlie had been sufficiently concerned about its structural integrity to have an engineer look over his design and run a few calculations.

The July afternoon Joe and I first heard about the engineer—Charlie having accepted Joe's dare-you invitation to help us cut and nail rafters—the architect came in for a lot of kidding. The day was very much Joe's. Cutting rafters is a complicated and unforgiving procedure, and Joe had shown up on time and armed with a detailed sketch indicating the precise location and angle of each of the four cuts each rafter needed: the ridge and tail cuts at each end—parallel to one another at a forty-five-degree angle to the rafter's edge—and the heel and seat cuts that form the "bird's mouth" where the rafter engages the top of the wall—a rectangular notch that in our case had to have a slightly different depth, or heel cut, on each rafter to account for the fact that our two side walls were not precisely parallel.

Joe had clearly done his homework, could even spout the formula for determining the length of a rafter: $\sqrt{run^2 + rise^2}$, in which the rise is the height of the gable and the run is the horizontal distance covered by each rafter, or one half the width of the building.

---

* This might explain why Vitruvius' definition of architecture included machines and timepieces as well as buildings; all were technologies devised by man to mediate his relationship to the natural world.

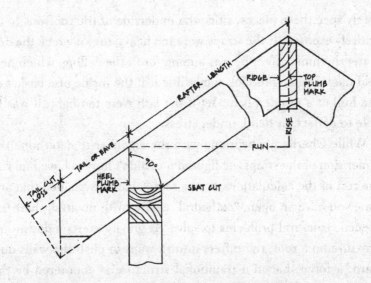

For his part, Charlie was feeling somewhat deflated after a punishing meeting with a client, and seemed in no shape to mix it up with a cocky carpenter who'd come equipped with enough geometry to frame a roof single-handed and who didn't see much point in architects to begin with.

"Charlie, just explain this to me," Joe began, gesturing with his big carpenter's square. "The building is only eight feet by thirteen, correct? It gets a roof that's framed with four-by-eight rafters and a ridge beam ten inches thick. *Plus* you're calling for two collar ties and a pair of king posts, all of which you want us to dowel together. So tell me: How can we *possibly* have anything to worry about structurally? This building's been designed for a *three*-hundred-year storm!"

Charlie managed a wan smile. He explained, somewhat sheepishly, that he'd needed to check with the engineer on the dimensions and spacing of the straps—the strips of wooden lath that run perpendicularly across the rafters to give us something to nail our shingles to. The fact that our rafters are a full thirty inches apart meant the lath would have to span an unusually great distance. Charlie had wanted to know the minimum dimensions he could safely spec these pieces, since the underside of the roof was to be entirely exposed. If the straps were too heavy, they'd wreck the delicate, rhythmic effect he was aiming for in the ceiling, which he'd told me was going to look something like the inside of a basket or the hull of a wooden boat. Yet if the lath were too light, it was liable to deflect, or bend, under stress.

While Charlie was working with the engineer to determine the dimension of the straps, he figured it couldn't hurt to have him run the rest of the calculations on the roof. Charlie explained that any time you have an open, "cathedral" ceiling with no attic, there are special structural problems to solve. As gravity exerts a downward pressure on a roof, the rafters in turn want to push the walls outward, a force that in a traditional structure is countered by the ceiling joists, which tie each pair of rafters together at the bottom, joining them in a taut triangle. But when the living space reaches directly up under the roof, these joists are eliminated, so either the walls have to be sturdy enough to withstand the outward thrust of the rafters or an occasional cross-tie beam must be provided to counteract it. It was Frank Lloyd Wright who pioneered such a ceiling, and it may well have been the novel structural and insulating problems it raised that caused some of his roofs to leak. Following Wright's example, Charlie wanted to give the interior of my building a pronounced sense of "roofness," one of those instances in architecture where expressing a structure seems, ironically, to complicate its construction.

"Anyway, you'll be happy to hear we've got nothing to worry about—the two cross-ties take care of our lateral stresses, and the king posts cut the weight carried by the ridge pole almost in half. And as far as those dowels are concerned, don't forget that in a storm you have upward forces working on a roof, too."

Joe and I both laughed; nothing about my building seemed in danger of blowing away. A few weeks before, as the frame was taking shape, I'd remarked to Charlie about how very heavy it looked.

"But it's not meant to be light," Charlie had protested. "This is your study, your library—it's an institution!" When I passed that one on to Joe, a look of concern swept over his face: "Mike, don't you think there's *another* kind of institution we should be talking to Charlie about?"

But there was nothing funny about the issue as far as Charlie was concerned. Charlie's nightmares, I knew, featured collapsing roofs and deflecting cantilevers. No doubt the fact that this particular design was being built by a crew consisting 50 percent of me made him even more nervous than usual. Out of the blue, Charlie would phone to reassure himself I was using galvanized nails in the frame; he'd heard about a house on Cape Cod that had simply crumpled to the ground one day, the salt air having rusted its common nails to dust. No doubt such worries disturb the sleep of all architects to one degree or another. When the massive concrete cantilevers of Fallingwater were being poured, Frank Lloyd Wright, delirious with fever at the time, was heard to mumble, "Too heavy! Too heavy!"*

"You two can laugh," Charlie said, "but I'm the one who's ultimately responsible, and it makes me sleep better knowing that an engineer has run all the calculations." He launched into a story he'd already told me twice before, about an opening-day bridge collapse in Tacoma. Joe chimed in with a few horror stories of his own, the sort of thing I imagine you could get your fill of in the bar at a convention of structural engineers, and by the time he got around to a fatal hotel atrium collapse in Kansas City, we were all feeling pretty good about our roof, about just how beefy it was going to be. While we talked, the three of us were lifting the chunky rafters into place, lining them up over the fin walls as best we could (our frame being, in Joe's cheerful new formulation, "too

---

* As it turned out he was nearer to the mark in his delirium than he had been in his calculations, because Fallingwater's cantilevers eventually did deflect.

hip to be square") and then toe-nailing them to the ridge beam above and wall plate below with (galvanized) twelve-penny nails almost as fat as pencils. We had all eight rafters securely in place before Charlie had to drive back to Cambridge, and the completed roof frame looked for all the world like a gigantic rib cage, its great fir bones wrapping themselves around a sheltered heart of space. Add to this skeleton a skin of cedar shingles, and you had the very kind of place where a body wouldn't mind riding out the storm of the century.

≡

It seems difficult if not impossible to avoid figurative language when talking about roofs, they're so evocative, so much more than the sum of their timbers and shingles and nails. To creatures who depend on them for their survival, it is perhaps inevitable that roofs are symbols of shelter as well as shelters themselves. Seen from afar or in a painting or movie, roofs also symbolize *us*—our presence in a landscape. Of course people have attached innumerable other meanings to roofs as well, and many of these meanings have changed over time. The traditional gable, for example, meant something very different after modernism than it did before.

Many of the important battles over style in architectural history can be seen as battles over roof types: the Gothic arch versus the classical pediment, the Greek Revival gable versus the Colonial saltbox, the international style flattop versus all of history's pitched roofs. In this century, the pitched roof became the most hotly contested symbol in all of architecture. Nothing did more to define modernist architecture than its adoption of the flat roof—and nothing did more to define postmodernism than its resurrection of the gable. Since then, architecture's avant-garde has sought to explode the very idea of a stable, dependable roof, violently "deconstructing" both the gable and the flattop. But the twentieth-century argument about roofs turns out to be about a lot more than that: it's really an argument about the very nature of architectural meaning, which seems to have undergone a thorough transformation in the last few years. I've come to think this transformation holds a clue to the disappearance of the old idea that architecture was somehow grounded in nature, as well as to the subsequent rise of the kind of literary architecture I had found in the pages of *Progressive Architecture*. You can get a good view of these developments up on the roof.

≡

"Starting from zero" was the rallying cry of modern architecture, and for the roof that meant banishing the gable, which the modern movement took as a key symbol of the architectural past—of everything musty and old and sentimental. Arguably the pitched roof (of which the gable is the most basic form) is architecture's first and most important convention—wasn't that the point of all those primitive-hut tales?—and under the modernist dispensation all conventions were to be tested against the standard of pure rationalism and function. The demonstrable fact that the pitched roof is *supremely* functional suggests that modernist rationalism sometimes took a backseat to modernist iconoclasm.

One of the aims of modern architecture was to rid the sprawling, many-gabled Victorian house of its many ghosts, all the historical encumbrances and psychological baggage that kept us from stepping out into the cleansing light and fresh air of the new century. In this sense modernist architecture was a therapeutic program. "If we eliminate from our hearts and minds all dead concepts in regard to the house," Le Corbusier wrote, "we shall arrive at the House Machine . . . healthy (and morally so, too) and beautiful in the same way that the working tools and instruments that accompany our existence are beautiful." In the modern view, the pitched roof was itself a "dead concept," but equally unhealthy were all those other dead concepts that got stored underneath the gable, in the attic. For there is where the ghosts of our past reside: the bric-a-brac and mementos that a lifetime collects; the love letters, photographs, and memories that clutter an attic and threaten to bear us back in time.

Modernism's program of psychological hygiene sought to rationalize everything about the house, to exorcise its ghosts and render it as unhaunted and transparent as a machine. Glass would supply the transparency, but it was the elimination of the pitched roof and its attic (along with the depths of the basement) that promised to vanquish the dead hand of the past, thereby helping to streamline the house's occupants for the challenge of the new age. Of course there were some who protested the wholesale housecleaning: Bachelard's *Poetics of Space* is an impassioned celebration of attics and basements and all those irrational but nevertheless powerfully symbolic places that modernism had banished from the house. People cannot dream in a "geometric cube," Bachelard complained. But then, that was the point. The irrational symbolic power of things like roofs and attics is precisely what made them so objectionable.

It's hard for us to imagine now just how powerful the taboo against gabled roofs in architecture was until very recently. I say "in architecture," because of course ordinary home buyers and commercial developers never really surrendered their attachment to pitched roofs, though modernism did manage to diminish the pitches on the vernacular roof, working like some powerful g-force to flatten the steep Victorian gable into the shallow hipped roofs found atop millions of suburban ranches. The architectural historian Vincent Scully writes in *The Shingle Style Today* that when he set out to build a house for himself in New Haven in 1950, "the model of reality in which I was imprisoned"—he had just completed his dissertation—"made it unthinkable to employ anything other than a flat roof . . ."

A dozen years later Robert Venturi single-handedly cracked open this model of reality and freed all the architects who'd been trapped inside it. He built a house for his mother in Chestnut Hill, Pennsylvania, that featured a gigantic, emphatic, in-your-face gable. The Vanna Venturi house, which was completed in 1964, proved to be the opening shot in architecture's postmodern revolution—"the biggest small building of the second half of the twentieth century," Scully has called it. Venturi has written that in 1964, even though there were a few single-slope shed roofs creeping back into architecture, the very act of designing a façade "where two slopes met to form a pediment contravened a taboo." At the time, his big front gable was "both too familiar and too old-fashioned, too rare and too outrageous."

What a revealing way to put it! For had Venturi's gable been *only* "too familiar and too old-fashioned," it would not have qualified as modern architecture. Instead of catching the eye of the Vincent Scullys of the world, the Vanna Venturi house would probably have been dismissed as revivalism—as something reactionary and nostalgic—or, worse, simply overlooked as a naïve vernacular building; after all, there had to have been a hundred thousand other pitched roofs erected in 1964. To count as modern architecture, Venturi's building had to be "rare and outrageous," too, and that it most certainly was.

For as anyone with eyes could see, there was something very peculiar about this particular gable. To begin with, it was on the long side of the house, which made it seem way too big—as if it had been exaggerated for effect, which of course it had. Then, right up at the top where the two slopes were supposed to meet, there was this odd space, a kind of gap tooth through which you could make out an oversized chimney rising several feet back from the façade. The gap made it appear as though there were nothing behind the façade; it flattened the gable out and made the whole house look more like a cardboard model of a house than a real, three-dimensional building. Venturi wanted to use a gable (what better ammunition for his assault on modernism?), but not one that could ever be mistaken for an "old-fashioned" gable. So he gave his gable a sharp ironic twist, exaggerating it and hollowing it out until it looked more like a comment on a gable than the thing itself. As Venturi himself puts it, "the pediment used in this fashion becomes a sign, a kind of representation . . ."

Venturi's use of the word "sign" to describe his roof, rather than, say, "symbol," is significant. Arguably his house in Chestnut Hill invented a whole new voice in which buildings might speak, and the shift from architectural symbols to signs is a key to that transformation. In using the word "sign," Venturi is drawing on the vocabulary of semiology, which holds that all cultural activities can be profitably read as systems of signs that are structured like languages. Semiologists, and structuralists after them, borrowed their terms from the turn-of-the-century Swiss linguist Ferdinand de Saussure, whose theories have by now reached far beyond linguistics to influence literary studies, the social sciences, art criticism, and even, thanks in no small part to Robert Venturi, modern architecture.

The relationship of a linguistic sign to the thing it signifies, Saussure maintained, is accidental; signs get their meanings not from the things in the world they refer to, but from the system of signs of which they are a part. That is why a certain combination of letters—*ng* is an often-cited example—can mean something in one language while remaining completely opaque in another. It follows that the choice of any sign is completely arbitrary, purely a social convention. In *Learning from Las Vegas*, Venturi's influential study of architectural meaning, a book that is steeped in semiology, he offers his own example of the "arbitrariness of the signifier": In the system of Chinese roads signs, green means "stop," and red means "go." Venturi encouraged architects to think of gables and columns and arches as signs too, elements as conventional as the letter combination *ng* or a green stop sign on a Chinese road.

In the years since Venturi built his mother's house and published his two seminal manifestos, it has become the conventional wisdom, at least among architecture's avant-garde, that architecture is a kind of language and that all its various elements—the gables and arches and columns, the axes and patterns of fenestration and materials—are best understood as conventions having less to do with the nature of the world or the human body or even the facts of construction than with the sign system, or language, of architecture itself. This was something radically new. Even modernists had paid pitched roofs and all the other symbols they detested the compliment of taking them seriously, treating them as if they actually had some weight in the world beyond architecture. Also quite new was the divorce Venturi was proposing between the imagery of a building and its underlying structure, a relationship upon which the modernists had sought to ground a whole aesthetic. By redefining a work of architecture as a "decorated shed"—an indifferent structure with signs on it—Venturi had driven a wedge between the meaning and the making of buildings.

The Vanna Venturi house was the first work of architecture built on the foundation of the new linguistic metaphor. Like the letter combination *ng*, the various elements of Venturi's house—its gable and windows, the arch over its entranceway—are meant to be understood chiefly in terms of the language of architecture. In fact Venturi wants to make sure we look no further: he deliberately designed the house to resemble a model so that it would be, in his words, "not real so much as denotative." The weightless, cardboard look, which has become a hallmark of postmodern architecture, is a way of announcing that the concrete Here of this building is less important than the abstract There of its signification; for Venturi and the countless postmodernists who followed his revolutionary example, the scrim of representation matters more than the reality behind it.

Thus the thin, abstract gable on the Vanna Venturi house has less to do with the world in which it rains and snows than with the increasingly hermetic world of architecture, which is in fact its true mise-en-scène. The space the building occupies is as much the space of images and information—of "discourse"—as it is the space of experience and place and the weather. Though its roof may well keep the rain off Mrs. Venturi's head, her son is anxious that we regard it primarily as a communications device, a sign referring us to, and commenting upon, other roofs in architecture— the pediments of the Greek temple; the long, dramatic gable on McKim, Mead, and White's shingle-style Low house in Bristol, Rhode Island; and, of course, every flattop in the modernist canon.

If this sounds like a lot of inside baseball, it is. In fact the Venturi house was completely opaque to me until I'd waded out into the ocean of commentary that has been written about it. And once I'd done my homework, I understood that reading is in fact an essential part of the "experience" of this house. (Just my luck!) Indeed, the Vanna Venturi house is the mother of all literary architecture, of every word-bound building I'd hurt my head on in *Progressive Architecture*. But was it also, my reading made me wonder, the mother of my building as well?

≡

At the same time I'd been scaling the intellectually slippery slope of Robert Venturi's famous roof in Chestnut Hill, back in Cornwall Joe and I were spending our Saturdays perched literally on top of my own, nailing down strips of lath in preparation for shingling. We'd made the lath out of two-by-fours cut lengthwise in half, then oiled them with wood preservative, since they were liable to come into contact with moist shingles; the oil raised the sweeping grain of the fir and made what had served as our foot- and hand-holds treacherously slick. My roof is exactly twice as steep as Venturi's (the ratio of its rise to run is 1:1, compared to his 1:2), and yet it was much easier to get a hold on, since whatever sense of precariousness I felt up there that summer owed more to gravity and the oiled lath (the wood preservative had the consistency of chicken fat) than cerebration. Not that there wasn't a fair amount of that, too. For in the speculative interludes provided by the pleasantly undemanding work of shingling, I found myself occupied with the question of just what, if anything, my anonymous gable roof owed to Venturi's famous roof, since that was the one that had rehabilitated gables in the eyes of the profession. Did my not-so-primitive hut fit under the larger roof of postmodernism Venturi had helped to erect?

When Charlie stopped by one afternoon late in August, I was up on the roof working by myself, nailing down the last couple of straps in preparation for shingling. After showing off the progress Joe and I had made since his last site inspection, I asked him whether or not he considered my building to be postmodern. I understood this was not a polite question. No architect ever likes to be pigeonholed, or to acknowledge a debt to another architect, at least to one not yet dead. I also knew that the postmodern label covered a lot of architecture Charlie couldn't stand.

"My knee-jerk reaction is, No, your building isn't at all postmodern." "Knee-jerk" suggested a more considered reaction might be on deck, so I persisted. But wasn't there something postmodern about his use of classical proportions? And didn't the pitch of the roof, along with the corner columns and the cornice, give the building a passing resemblance to a Greek temple—exactly the sort of reference a postmodernist might make?

"Well, in that sense, yes, I *guess* . . . Oh, I don't know—" Charlie hates to find himself in even the most shallow theoretical waters. But after flailing around for a moment, he realized the only way back to shore was to start swimming. "Okay, look. To the extent that postmodernism made it okay to use historical elements again, I suppose you could say this is a postmodern building. And I guess I *do* think of it as a kind of temple. But it's not like I went and arbitrarily stuck a classical temple top on an office building out on Route 128!" He was referring to a Robert A.M. Stern building near Boston.

"So then is it a question of attitude?"

"Of conviction, yes. Look, an architect can employ a historical reference in an ironic or mannerist way, which is what I think of postmodernists as doing, or you use it because you think there's still something great about it, that it still has some value in a particular context. Those straps are a perfect example."

As we were talking, I was applying a second coat of chicken fat to the lath with an old paintbrush. Charlie's plans had called for the straps, which were spaced about five inches apart, to extend several inches beyond the first and last rafter, creating a reveal that had the effect of adding dentils to the façade of the building—another classical detail. Named for the teeth they resemble, dentils are the small square blocks that appear in series beneath the roofs of Greek temples, either directly above the cornice or along the slope of the pediment.

Charlie explained that the dentil is one of several classical ornaments that the Greeks derived from the timber framing on which they modeled their architecture; dentils were inspired by the exposed tips of the lath used to support the roofing material—which was precisely what the ones on my building were going to do.

"Now, a card-carrying postmodernist might use dentils too, but he'd do it in such a way that they were clearly mannerist or iconographic. They'd be purely and obviously decorative, for starters—pasted on, not structural. And then he'd either use lots and lots of really tiny dentils, or a handful of gigantic ones, to make absolutely clear the reference was playful or ironic. He'd probably want to paint them, too, for the added emphasis.

"But look at the straps on your roof. This is not a skin job. This is not irony. Those are *real* dentils! Oh, sure, they're a classical reference, too. But the reason I used dentils on this roof is because they still happen to work—they'll do a good job holding up our shingles, and explaining how our roof works. They're still alive, is what I guess I'm trying to say."

Charlie pulled a shingle from one of the bundles stacked on the floor and brought it to his nostrils. "Don't you love the smell of fresh cedar? I could just about eat this stuff." He passed the shingle to me as if it were the cork from a bottle of wine.

"Very often architects seem to be afraid to just come out and say they like something, they think they've got to take it back a little. So they'll use some element they like—these dentils, say—but they'll do it ironically as a way of protecting themselves. I suppose it's partly a matter of audience: Is your audience your client, or is it really New York and L.A. and the magazines? Because if that's who it is, then you're going to want to somehow announce you're a sophisticated, postmodern guy, that all this is just theater, instead of being willing to come out and say, 'This is *not* theater. It's here, it's real, and I happen to like it.'

"So does that make me a postmodernist or not?"

Yes and no, I decided later. It seemed as though the postmodern movement had opened a door through which a lot of people like Charlie might slip, under the cover of their more ironically inclined colleagues. What separated the two groups was their demeanor as much as anything else. Charlie had seized the license offered by postmodernism, but he hadn't bothered with the attitude that was supposed to go with it, the small print of pastiche on the back.

Charlie wasn't the only one. Out beyond the increasingly rarefied world of academic architecture, there didn't seem to be many other people paying attention to the small print, either. Postmodern architects might wield their historical reference in the correct ironic spirit, but how many people outside of architecture were really getting it? Because if somebody hadn't read the accompanying texts, and didn't know enough to spot the cardboard, he was apt to miss the signs for the irony exit and find himself driving shamelessly down the road of "nostalgia" (perhaps the dirtiest word in architecture today), reveling in the unself-conscious pleasures of old-fashioned pitched roofs and divided-light windows and stone façades. Right here lies an important reason for postmodernism's success (another is the fact that faux tends to be cheap): The architects might be selling signs, but the corporate patrons and the individuals commissioning postmodern buildings were often buying the old-fashioned, beloved, and sorely missed symbols.*

But historicist architecture was only one current released by postmodernism, even if it was the most visible and popular one. Having freed architecture from its traditional obligations to space and structure and symbolism, postmodernism also opened the way to a series of increasingly radical experiments in formalism. These aloof, relentlessly abstract buildings may have looked quite different from Venturi's, but their designers shared with him the conviction that architecture was a language; they just used different vocabularies to say different things. No longer driven by the exigencies of program or site or client or material or method of construction, the architect was now free as a sculptor, poet, or literary theorist, and he could enlist any set of metaphors or intellectual vocabulary he liked to drive his design. This might be architectural history, but it could just as easily be Boolean algebra, Chomskyan

---

* Something similar happened to modernism: What had been conceived as a radical, antibourgeois movement was rapidly transformed into the preferred style—the very logo— of corporate America, testament to capitalism's astounding power to co-opt even its sternest challengers. And so an aesthetic that grew out of European socialism, an architecture inspired by factories and worker housing projects, ended up producing elegant settings for power lunches on Park Avenue.

linguistics, inside jokes, conceptualism, cubism, pop culture, and, of course, deconstruction.

Peter Eisenman, whose own career describes an arc passing through a succession of these isms, is largely responsible for bringing this last and supposedly most subversive intellectual vocabulary to architecture. In the same way that Jacques Derrida sought to identify and then "deconstruct" a series of central metaphysical concepts in Western culture—humanism, phallocentrism, presence, truth—Eisenman and his colleagues set about deconstructing what they took to be architecture's own set of fundamental assumptions. The big four were shelter, aesthetics, structure, and meaning. Also ripe for deconstruction were all those other things about buildings people take for granted: that form had some organic relationship to function, that inside was intrinsically different than outside, that right side up was the way you wanted a building to be, that the roof went on top. Derrida had attacked writers and philosophers for borrowing metaphors of solidity and presence from buildings; now the architects were going the great philosopher one better, attacking the solidity and presence of the buildings themselves.*

Beginning in the 1970s Eisenman designed a series of houses that "attempted to destabilize the idea of home"—apparently another dubious social construction. Perhaps the most famous of these houses to actually get built (most didn't) was House VI, which happens to be in the town where I live. While I was roofing my own building, I read an article in the local paper about the travails of its owners and phoned them to ask if I could come by and see their famous house. The visit gave me my closest encounter

---

* As for Venturi himself, he often seemed shocked and dismayed by some of the architecture his revolution had spawned, occasionally playing the role of Danton to Peter Eisenman's Robespierre. "If you're lucky," he recently wrote, "you live long enough to see the bad results of your good ideas." He has described deconstructivist architecture as "sculpture with a resented roof."

with some of the astonishing feats of which architects are capable once they've put aside their usual concerns about client, site, materials, structure, place, and time. It took me deep into the very heart of architectural unreality.

Pulling into the driveway on a hot summer afternoon, my first impression of the house was that it resembled some sort of spiny gray-and-white spaceship hovering several feet above the lawn. The architect had recessed the foundation from the intersecting planes that comprise the house's walls, and this made it appear as though the building never quite touches down on its site. There's no façade to speak of, and no visible means of entry. Eisenman's idea, I read later, was to overturn the usual relationship between inside and outside, in which the façade of a building inaugurates the process by which we make sense of it; here, sense-making (such as it is) was deliberately frustrated until you were inside.

Eventually I located the entrance, a gunmetal steel fire door hidden around a corner, and met the Franks, a friendly couple in their early sixties (Dick is a food photographer, Suzanne an architectural historian) who appear to have done more than their fair share for the glory of contemporary architecture. Suzanne has written an illuminating book about the house, *Peter Eisenman's House VI: The Client's Response,* that details both the satisfactions and the trials of living in a work of art. The book recounts the time Eisenman called to say that he was bringing Philip Johnson over to see the house. Apprehensive about the great man's reaction, Eisenman asked the Franks if they wouldn't mind removing the baby's crib from the house so Johnson could experience the building in its pristine form; the Franks obligingly put their baby's crib out on the lawn. There's a picture of Eisenman in the book, visiting the construction site; the architect looks like the hippest professor you had in college: bushy, well fed, bespectacled, and smoking a pipe.

Asked at the time why he took what appeared to be a cavalier approach to his clients' needs, Eisenman patiently explained that his goal was to "shake them out of those needs." That may explain why the single bathroom is accessible only by walking through the Franks' bedroom. Or why, in deference to the complex geometrical system that governs the design, the floor of the tiny master bedroom has a gaping slot cut through it in such a way as to rule out a double bed. (There's one need the architect had presumably shaken his clients out of.) One column, its location dictated not by the structure but by the geometry, awkwardly divides the dining area in such a way as to frustrate conversation at the dinner table.

As for the roof, it too has been "destabilized," and in more ways than one. Originally punctuated by flat "windows," the roof is designed to look all but indistinguishable from a wall. This is apparently because the architect wanted to invert the "conventional" relationship of roof and wall, as well as up and down; there's also an upside-down staircase suspended over the dinner table, and a column suspended from the roof that fails to reach all the way to the ground. In theory the house should look pretty much the same if you were to rotate it in space. But the flat, fenestrated roof leaked so badly that the frame of the house rotted out within just a few years of construction.

When the Franks decided that they would replace a section of their flat roof with a gently sloped one, Eisenman, an old friend, publicly attacked them for spoiling the lines of his design, and the Franks found themselves accused of "cultural vandalism" in the pages of *Art in America*. A few years later the Franks drained their savings to have the house almost entirely rebuilt. This time they were able to work out a few compromises with Eisenman, who signed off on conventional bubble skylights, a slight pitch in the roof, and even a double bed that bridges the slot in the floor.

After I'd signed the guest book, adding my name to an impressive roster of some of architecture's leading lights, I thanked Suzanne and Dick for their hospitality. On the drive home it occurred to me that the best way to understand the Franks' strange home was as a kind of antiprimitive hut for our time. For House VI offers the precise negative image of the old hut ideal, an alternative myth that denies point by point everything about architecture that the canonical hut had claimed about nature and structure and material and shelter.

The primitive hut had said that the forms and meaning of architecture were derived from nature; House VI was a virtuoso display of architecture as the pure product of culture—of whatever sign system the architect chose to deploy. The primitive hut said that architectural structure was an expression of its materials and how it was made; both the structure and materials of House VI were perfectly silent; there's no way to tell that there's a conventional balloon frame under the building's "dematerialized" surface, a surface that at various times has been clad in stucco and acrylic. The purpose of the primitive hut was to shelter us, to minister to our needs; House VI seeks to destabilize the notion of shelter, to shake us out of our needs.

In fact these two contending dreams of architecture were equally unreal; this much now seemed clear. To claim that nature was the source of all architectural truth was just as absurd as the postmodernist's claim that architecture rested on no foundation whatsoever, that it was culture all the way down. No doubt the truth lay somewhere in-between. The old hut designers and the new ones, I understood after visiting House VI, are equally deft cartoonists of what is surely a more mixed reality.

Eisenman and architects like him are hell-bent on liberating architecture from every conceivable earthly bond: from program, function, history, home, the body, and nature itself. It is, to be sure, a daring project, provocative as art, or philosophy. It's a poignant one too, for as the revenge of nature, and client, on House VI suggests, it is probably doomed. Looking around House VI, trying to make sense of its geometrical inversions, of the elegant There its architect wants me to dwell on, I found my attention kept snagging on the banal, neglected Here of the place: the cracks in the paint job on the upside-down staircase; the way my head grazed a beam as I climbed the right-side-up one; the dust balls collecting in the corners of the slots in the walls; the smell of the Franks' spaniels; the mildew already starting to stain the space-age acrylic that had been sprayed on the exterior when it was rebuilt. Nothing more than the usual wear and tear, but here it leapt out rudely, offering what seemed like a kind of rebuke. What it made me understand is that House VI was never so perfect, never so true to itself, as the day before the day the Franks moved in. Or perhaps you have to go back further still, to the day it was first drawn. Ever since, the house has been in a steady process of decline, as the ordinary frictions of reality and everyday life, the dogs and the people and the rain, have taken their incremental toll, sullying Eisenman's dream of pure architectural Idea. Architecture might be done with nature, but the experience of House VI, now on its third roof, suggests that nature will never be done with architecture.

≡

I know, I promised I wasn't going to make too much here of leaky roofs. But I was thinking about leaks all the time that summer, since so much of our work on the roof was aimed at preventing them. Charlie had sent me a brochure issued by the Cedar Bureau, a trade organization to which he accords an almost papal authority. The bureau advises builders on the correct handling of cedar shingles (by far the best kind for wood roofs), and we followed their counsel to the letter. From the bureau we learned such things as the proper grade of cedar to use on a roof, the best kind of nails to secure them with, the optimal gap to leave between adjacent shingles (they need room to expand in the heat), how to overlap all the seams on one course with the shingles of the next, and precisely how much of every shingle should be exposed to the weather (no more than 5½″ on a roof of our pitch).

There was a lot to it, which is why Joe and I found ourselves taking far greater pains with our roof than with, say, our walls. Though the whole building was to be skinned in shingles, we were using white cedar on the walls and red on the roof; red was considerably more expensive, but you wanted its superior stability and weather resistance on the roof. Everything I was learning about how to make a roof impressed on me that the roof was, well, different. You couldn't possibly work on one and still seriously entertain the idea that roofs and walls might be handled in the same manner. From up here, that was strictly a drafting-table conceit. Am I starting to sound like a cranky carpenter ragging on ivory-tower architects? Maybe, but the work of roofing does little to encourage a belief in the arbitrariness of roofs, or their deep linguistic nature.

Joe would watch me carefully as I lapped my shingles, letting me know when a seam in one course edged too close to the seam in the course below. He taught me how to notch the handle of my hammer 5½″ from the end; this way I merely had to flip the hammer over to set each shingle's proper exposure to the weather, instead of having to reach for my tape. (Working up on the roof, you want as few tools to worry about dropping as possible.) He taught me the proper way to cut a shingle: how you scored the shingle with a utility knife, then broke it cleanly along the grain. And he taught me how to cultivate randomness in the widths of my shingles by reaching into the stack without looking. Shingling, Joe would travel methodically across one face of the roof as if it were an ear of corn, then move up a course and return, shingling his way in the opposite direction. At first I moved haltingly across the roof's opposite slope, but after a few courses I absorbed the rhythm of the work—reach for a shingle, slap it down on the one below, adjust its exposure with my handle, flip the hammer, nail it down, reach for another—and began to match his swift and easy pace.

The shingles themselves, colored an earthy red shading to tobacco, surprised me with their inconsequentiality. At the business end they were less than half an inch thick, and they dwindled to paper at the other. It was nothing to break one of them in half. Yet layered and woven with enough care, these aromatic slips of cedar made a sturdy shelter, could withstand even a New England nor'easter. It wasn't until I'd handled a few hundred of them that I fully appreciated the design of Charlie's roof, the way he'd underscored with his fat rafters and fine lath the delicate weave of wood that a shingle roof is. Building it, you knew this was a roof designed by someone who'd probably once done some roof work himself, someone who had given a lot of thought to what a cedar shingle is.

The architect Louis Kahn used to talk about interrogating his materials in order to learn what they "wanted to be"—that is, what the distinctive nature of a material suggested should be done with it:

> You say to brick, "What do you want, brick?" Brick says to you, "I like an arch." If you say to brick, "Arches are expensive, and I can use a concrete lintel over an opening. What do you think of that, brick?" Brick says, "I like an arch."

The stuff we make our buildings out of—our bricks and cedar shingles, our concrete and stucco and even plastic—is perhaps the first way that nature expresses itself in our architecture. Working attentively with their materials can draw the architect and builder into a kind of dialogue with the material world; you learn a lot about a shingle—and about red cedar—watching how it responds to your handling. Of course the architect doesn't have to honor his materials in the way Kahn describes; he's free in designing to interrogate a philosophical conceit rather than a brick or a shingle, or to strive for a "dematerialized" look in his surfaces. But he probably runs certain risks in doing so. Sooner or later a stain will expose the materiality of his stucco or plastic, if the rain doesn't undermine it first. Try as it might, no building ever transcends the stuff it's made of.

Materials are so essential to our physical experience of a place that to disregard them—to ignore the coldness of steel, the dumb strength of concrete, the sympathy of wood, whose temperature never startles—is to throw away a great deal of architecture's expressive power. Is the nature of that power linguistic? Certainly my shingles signified specific things to my mind ("New England," for example), but they also addressed my senses more directly, with their aroma, their delicateness, with the impression they gave my hands of wanting to be layered and woven for strength. It seemed to me you wouldn't seriously argue that architecture was a language unless you'd forgotten the specific heft of a cool brick, or the smell of fresh cedar warmed in the afternoon sun. The reality and presence and Hereness of these things, the sense they give us of wanting to do one thing and not another, exert a worldly pressure on building that an architect would have to go out of his way to ignore. As for a builder, he wouldn't even think to try.

While we shingled, Joe and I talked, mainly about "ice dams." Ice dams are probably the most serious threat facing a roof in the northern latitudes. It seems that when snow on a roof is melted by the heat radiating upward from the interior of a building, meltwater streams down the slope until it reaches the much-colder eaves, where it's apt to freeze again, building up in a heavy block along the lower edge of the roof. This is why Charlie had spec'd two-by-six planking under the first three feet of shingles, instead of the relatively light straps we were using higher up.

But weight is apparently not the only danger an ice dam presents. A thick one will block the flow of meltwater in the spring and actually force it to back up the slope of the roof and then under the shingles, where it is liable to infiltrate the building and drip onto one's head. One reason roofs are steeper in snowier climates is to prevent ice dams, since a steep roof will shed precipitation more quickly than a shallow one; the steeper a roof's pitch, the less likely it is meltwater will travel back up its slope. Perched near the peak of my own roof, holding on to the slicked straps for dear life, I had the testimony of my own body to these facts, as the muscles in my legs registered the slope's distinct wish to shed my weight.

The easiest way for an architect to avoid problems with his roof is to pay more attention to vernacular practice. Vernacular roofs—most of which happen to be pitched, the precise pitch varying with the latitude and local snowfall—reflect the experience of thousands of builders over hundreds of years; they represent a successful adaptation to a given environment, a good fit between the human desire to keep dry and the predictable behavior of water and wood under specific circumstances. There's nothing inherently wrong with attempting something more adventurous, but, as in the case of an evolutionary mutation, there's a greater risk that the novel design will fail. When Frank Lloyd Wright declared that "If the roof doesn't leak the architect hasn't been creative enough," he had a point. There seems to be an inherent tension between architectural novelty and sound construction.*

The vernacular roof suggests another way that nature finds its way into architecture, sanctioning one solution and rendering others suspect. After long trial and error, builders discovered that the pitched roof worked best at keeping the rain out of buildings built in wood. So it means something to say that, under certain circumstances, a pitched roof is more "natural" than some other kind—that is, more in keeping with the way this world we've been given seems to work. And we can say this without having to say anything categorical about "nature." All we're saying is that, *whatever* nature really is, it seems to behave in one way in the case of a pitched

---

* To clients who complained about roof leaks, Frank Lloyd Wright's stock response was, "That's how you can tell it's a roof." The owner of (flat-roofed) Fallingwater used to refer to his house as "Rising Mildew" and a "seven-bucket building."

roof, and another in the case of a flat one. We may not know nature directly, as the deconstructors never tire of reminding us, but we do have long experience of what works and what doesn't work in nature. My own hard-won experience of right angles, for example, has convinced me that, whatever the deconstructivists might think, ours is indeed a ninety-degree world. Lloyd Kahn, once a leading advocate of dome-shaped houses, came to a similar conclusion after actually building and living in one:

> What's good about 90-degree walls: they don't catch dust, rain doesn't sit on them, easy to add to; gravity, not tension, holds them in place. It's easy to build in counters, shelves, arrange furniture, bathtubs, beds. *We* are 90 degrees to the earth.

The subject of leaky roofs also suggested to me that there might be certain architectural conventions that "mean" in a less arbitrary way than signs do. Geographers tell us they can infer the climate of a region from the steepness of the roofs found there; the steeper the slope of the typical roof, the more snow the region receives. The pitch of a vernacular roof may be conventional, but it is not arbitrary; it represents something more than caprice or fashion or a "social construction." Put another way, the roof derives at least one of its meanings—the one about climate—not from the agreement of a group of people in architecture or the field of geography, but from certain facts of nature. Its form is less like a combination of letters in a language than a body part or camouflage device that, far from being arbitrary, exhibits a specific fitness to its environment.

Even Robert Venturi and Peter Eisenman would grant this much to nature: Architecture's roofs should not leak. Oh yes, and one other thing: gravity—architecture has got to stand up too. Eisenman allows that a building must work as structure (it should stand up) and shelter (it should stay dry)—though he insists it needn't *look* like it stands up and stays dry. But after that, anything goes. Venturi adds that, since anyone can make a shed stand up and stay dry, the really good minds should occupy themselves with the signs and ornamentation.

And this is how big-time architecture is practiced today, at least by stars like Eisenman and Venturi. Read the credits on important new buildings and you will invariably find two architectural firms listed: one you've heard of, and another you probably haven't. For example, on the Wexner Center for the Arts in Columbus, Ohio, perhaps Peter Eisenman's most famous actually constructed building, he shares credit with an obscure local firm by the name of Richard Trott & Partners. The famous architect's firm will give a building its signature look—deconstructivist, postmodern, whatever—and then a second, unheralded firm is called in to flesh out the design in such a way as to make sure the building will stand up and stay dry and pass muster with the building inspector. In effect, the whole leaky roof problem has been subbed out.

As this division of architectural labor suggests, the work of construction and the work of design have drifted some distance apart, and you can't help but wonder (especially when you're groping for a reliable foothold on a slicked roof) whether this gulf might not help explain the increasingly abstract and literary quality of so much contemporary architecture, not to mention a great many leaky roofs. The history of architecture is the history of the widening of that gulf, from the time when master builders designed and built buildings themselves; to the Renaissance, when architects began designing buildings but left decisions about construction and ornament to craftsmen on site; to our own time, when celebrated architects concentrate on the skin of the building, the details of construction fall to local engineering and design firms, and the craftsman, the one with his hands on the thing itself, has been reduced to an unconsulted laborer. It stands to reason that the greater an architect's distance from the actual work of making buildings, the more likely he would be to embrace what Venturi has called an "architecture of communication over space."

By now, a tendency to emphasize signs at the expense of space, or physical experience, is probably built into the way contemporary architecture gets practiced and judged. The architect is bound to stress There in favor of Here when There is where the architect works. The arena in which a great deal of the work of architecture is performed today is on paper: in the articles and photographs used to disseminate and comment upon buildings and chart the rise and fall of architects' careers. Building buildings is no longer even a prerequisite to a successful architectural career, as Peter Eisenman, John Hejduk, Robert Venturi, and a great many other current and former paper architects can testify. (Eisenman is probably right to suggest, as he once did, that the actual building of House VI was all but incidental to the project.) In the case of buildings that do get built, since it is very often not the client's but the media's opinion that really matters, architects will naturally tend to emphasize those elements in their designs that can be communicated effectively in the relevant media, and these are inevitably going to have more to do with two-dimensional signs than with three-dimensional space, more with images and information than with the tactile qualities of materials and the experience of space. This kind of work has acquired a name: "magazine architecture." Of course, it never rains in magazines.

≡

Rain and gravity: Are these really the only facts of nature architecture has to worry about? Is structure and shelter as far as the architect's obligation to reality goes? For a long time it seemed to me that this might in fact be the case; that Venturi and Eisenman had driven nature into a very tight corner indeed, and, after taking account of those two irreducible basics they could safely ignore it. The rest was all culture and fashion and taste: Anything goes. I couldn't see any way out of this tight corner—until, that is, I chanced to talk to Charlie about a somewhat unusual commission he was working on the summer I raised my roof.

It was, of all things, a design for a birdhouse, and what he told me about it made me wonder if the place of nature in architecture might not be more extensive and subtle than a postmodernist would think. Specifically, Charlie was designing a wood duck house for a man who had built a pond to which he was eager to attract wildlife. The wood duck is a threatened species that is apparently quite choosy about its nesting sites. Charlie started from the assumption that his client was in some sense a duck, even though he understood he had to design a structure that would please the eye of his human (and fee-paying) client as well. So he spent a couple of afternoons at the library of the comparative zoology department at Harvard, learning all he could about the needs and nesting habits of *Aix sponsa*.

To succeed, Charlie's little building would not only have to stand up and shed water (the postmodern shed's bottom line), but must exhibit a whole series of other characteristics necessary to win the attention and ensure the comfort of wood ducks—characteristics that don't fit under the rubric of ornament; no "decorated shed" was likely to do the trick here. The entrance, for example, had to be four inches in diameter, an aperture large enough to admit the female but not the male; this is an arrangement a nesting wood duck evidently insists upon. The opening should be several inches deep as well, to prevent a raccoon from reaching in to snatch the eggs. Beyond that, the interior needed to be a well-ventilated vertical space dropping down below the entrance tunnel. Lastly, the house had to be sited either directly over a pond or no more than a few feet from the shore, so that the mother could conduct her ducklings to the safety of open water soon after their emergence from the nest.

The basic idea, as Charlie explained it to me, was to recreate the characteristics of a fairly large woodpecker hole in a dead, hollowed-out tree near a pond or in a swamp—the wood duck's natural habitat. Charlie was free to design the building to look any way he wanted—vernacular, postmodern, deconstructivist, whatever— but in a few key respects it had better remind a wood duck of a woodpecker hole in a tree or no wood duck would ever come near it. What struck me as significant about this was that Charlie was attempting not to *fool* the wood duck, who would understand perfectly well that this gabled house on stilts (it wound up looking a lot like a Charlie Myer house) was neither a tree nor a woodpecker hole, but to somehow *evoke* those things. In a sense, Charlie's wood duck house was an acknowledged piece of artifice designed to symbolize the wood duck's natural habitat; as one thing that referred to another, you might say it was a kind of duck metaphor.

I know; I'm talking about ducks. Yet Charlie's wood duck house made me appreciate that, even to a duck, the landscape brims with meaning. Certain formations in it imply certain qualities: To a duck, a deep hole set high over water connotes safety and convenience. This suggests a couple of things that seemed at least potentially relevant to human architecture. Meaning is not always a function of language or even communication; to wood ducks at least (who by the way can also communicate among themselves in the usual manner, by quacking), the things of this world are not mute but sometimes speak to a creature directly, carrying meanings of shelter, of danger, of nourishment, of sexual opportunity—all meanings that don't depend on a sign system or culture of any kind. The meaning of a four-inch hole set high over water is the product not of an agreement among wood ducks—of cultural consensus—but of the species's evolution. It came into the world whenever it was that wood ducks first figured out that, given the shape and size of a wood duck body and certain facts about the species's reproduction, this particular formation denoted a superior shelter; in the case of this species, "symbolism"—perhaps even in some sense "taste"—is a by-product of survival: of what works.

And yet there's no denying the existence of countless symbols and conventions that *are* entirely arbitrary and cultural. Even Charlie's wood duck house featured symbols that almost certainly meant nothing to a wood duck, that were strictly part of a system of signs, a language you had to learn. There were a series of details, for example, that signified a human home: the gable roof, a trio of tiny windows along each side, and some ornament around the entrance that heightened the sense of ceremony there. These things were obviously directed not at ducks but at people.

What this suggests is that very different orders of symbolism can coexist in a building. Some symbols are patently just as arbitrary as the postmodernists say. How else to account for the fact that, in the first half of the nineteenth century, great white fluted columns on the front of an American house symbolized republican virtue in one part of the country and a slave-holding aristocracy in another? Had Charlie put fluted white columns on the façade of his duck house, they would have been nothing more than a sign, as meaningless as *ng* to a duck and, for that matter, to anybody else not versed in that particular human cultural system. So how could you have it both ways: fluted columns that were wholly arbitrary and four-inch holes (or, closer to home, pitched roofs) that were clearly fitted to the facts of nature? The birdhouse suggested a simple hypothesis: Maybe architecture speaks in more than one voice, the first grounded in meanings at least partly given by nature and another trafficking in meanings determined mainly by culture.

≡

Soon after formulating this hypothesis, I found some human backing for it right in my own human building. Joe and I had finished shingling our roof, capping it at the peak with two well-caulked, -glued, and -screwed-together cedar ridge boards, and we'd turn our attention to closing in the rest of the building. We nailed four-by-eight sheets of three-quarter-inch plywood to the frame, whole ones first, and then smaller sections cut around the rough openings where the windows and the door would go. A layer of house wrap and then shingles would later be stapled and nailed, respectively, onto the plywood sheathing to complete the building's walls.

No other single step in the whole construction process had so swift and dramatic an impact on the building as the nailing up of that plywood cladding. After just a couple of hours of work, the building, which before had stood open to the weather on all sides, had acquired a skin and with that an interior; what had been merely a wooden diagram of a structure was suddenly a house. Until now, Joe and I would always "enter" the structure willy-nilly, stepping in between any two studs wherever we pleased. But as soon as we had nailed up the last sheet of plywood, the only way in was through the door.

I tried it first, approaching and entering the building the way we were meant to, and the experience took me aback. Now that the building was clad, its bulk blocked the view down to the pond as you came around the big rock and turned into the site. What I saw before me was the body of the building to my left and the mass of the boulder on my right, two hulking forms separated only by a triangular wedge of space that closed down to a point where house and rock almost touched. Stepping through the narrow doorway, beneath the overhanging eave (inches above my head), then under the low cornice plank and between the two fin walls, the sense of constricted space suggested by the narrow wedge of ground outside seemed momentarily to intensify. But as soon as I had arrived inside and stood there on the upper landing, I could feel the space begin to relax around me.

Now I turned to my right and stepped down into the main room, drawn by the flood of light and landscape coming in through the big rough opening on the west wall where my desk would go. Two things seemed to happen simultaneously as I stepped down into the main space. This bright sense of broad prospect all but exploded right in front of me—the shimmery pond framed now not only by the oak and ash outside, but by the thick, vertical corner posts inside as well—and the weight of the ceiling, this canopy of shingles layered like so many leaves against its frame of lath and rafters, was lifted right off my shoulders as if I'd been suddenly relieved of a heavy winter coat. I noticed how, on turning into the light-filled opening beneath the lifting-off ceiling, you could not help but let out a chestful of air, as your body perceived and then entered into this most welcome release of space going on all around it.

And yet not *all* around it, for this was no glass house, after all. On either side of me an arm's length away stood these two tall, thick, companionable walls that lent the space an unmistakable sense of refuge; I felt as though I captained this broad prospect from the safety of a sturdy enclosure. The tall walls so near at hand did something else too. They gave the building a pronounced trajectory, funneling the space coming down from the hillside behind it straight through this stepping-down wooden chute (through *me*, it almost seemed, standing directly in its path) and then out again, firing it between the trees and down into the pond below. There was something buoying about this, in the way the prospect said "Ahead!" and seemed to join the two senses of that word—prospect as seeing and prospect as opportunity. The building's interior seemed to underscore, or re-present, certain qualities of the landscape outside it: the powerful flow of chi running through it that I'd sensed back when I sited it, the delicateness of the overhanging canopy (reproduced in the leafy shingles and boughlike rafters), the counterpoised senses of prospect and refuge. Coming in from outside, these qualities of the site seemed more available, not less.

So here it was, this place of my own that I'd been working on for so long, and now I could feel it working on me. And "feel" was the right word for it too, for my experience of the room was a matter of so much more than just the eye; sure, the view was a big part of it (and the easiest to describe), but the experience of the space was at least as much a matter of the shoulders, of whatever that whiskery sense is that allows us to perceive the walls around us even in the dark. Even with my eyes shut tight I know I could have sensed that constriction of space followed by its sudden release, my brainstem performing some ancient animal calculus on the sense data streaming in, measuring the slight but perceptible changes in the properties of the air, subtle swings in its temperature and acoustics, even in the shifting scents of the different woods all around me. Our vocabulary for describing the work of the senses may be impoverished (one reason, perhaps, they don't get much play in the architectural treatises), but that doesn't mean the senses aren't always at it, giving shape to our sense of place, making the experience of space just that: a fully fledged *experience,* something greater than the sum of what you can read about or glean from the photographs in a magazine.

Joe was outside, gathering up his tools and getting ready to go, when I called him in to check out the new room. Plainly it worked on him too, because he gave a tremendous smile of satisfaction as he stepped down into the room and drank in the view. "Cool" was as much of an observation as he managed at first, and then: "It feels like I'm standing in a wheelhouse. On the bridge of the Mothership Organic! Mike, I think we built a goddamn boat." And there was definitely something to that. The ceiling did recall the ribbed hull of a sailboat, and the walls and windows left no doubt as to which way the prow lay, but what really made you feel that this might be the bridge of a ship was the sense of command you felt standing at the window, riding high over the landscape spread out before you, a fine, beneficent breeze of space (of chi?) at your back.

Perhaps what makes the experience of space so difficult to describe is that it involves not only a complex tangle of sense information (hard enough to sort out by itself) but also the countless other threads supplied by memory and association. As soon as you've begun to register the sensory data, the here-and-now-ness of the place, there arrives from somewhere else all the other rooms and landscapes it summons up—and in this particular case a couple of boats (and perhaps a tree house) as well. Even so, describing the experience of this room now, while it is still not much more than a thin shell of space, is probably as easy as it's ever going to get, for as Joe and I add to it the layers of finish and furnishings and trim, each carrying its own valence of memory and allusion, the complexity of the experience will only thicken. Here right now was the space of my building, as plain and fresh as it would ever be.

And what it helped me to understand is that space is not mute, that it does in fact speak to us, and that we respond to it more directly, more viscerally, than all the cerebral, left-brained talk about signs and conventions would have us think. I would venture, in fact, that we respond to it rather more like a wood duck than a deconstructionist. For whatever else you can say about it, the experience of coming into my building for the first time was not foremost a literary or semiological experience, a matter of communication. This is not to say that the experience wasn't rich with meanings and layered with symbols; it was, but the meanings and symbols were of a different order than the ones the architectural theorists talk about: no key was required to unlock their meaning.

≡

Well, actually there *is* one key needed to unlock the experience of this room, though it is not a textual key and it is a key all of us possess. I mean, of course, the human body, without which the experience of the room as I have described it would be meaningless. For only a body like our own (upright, and of more or less the same scale) could have fully registered the pleasing sequence of constriction and release I felt upon walking into the building or the expectant forward trajectory I'd sensed standing at the window, or been moved by the sense of prospect and refuge created by the juxtaposition of those thick walls and big windows—the window exactly wide enough to fill your field of vision completely, the walls almost close enough to give a reassuring tap.

So you don't have to take my word for it, or think my building unique in this regard, let me offer another, more well-known example: Grand Central Station, in Manhattan. As an architectural space, Grand Central is of course loaded with signs, literal as well as semiotic, having to do with the significance of arrival and departure, the rich symbolism of a railroad station in the heart of a great city, the whole complex of social meanings woven into that great cosmopolitan thrum. But anyone who has ever strode through this space recognizes that it works on us at a very different level as well. This is how J. B. Jackson describes it in an essay called "The Imitation of Landscape":

> . . . to the average man the immediate experience of Grand Central is neither architectural nor social; it is sensory. He passes through a marvelous sequence; emerging in a dense, slow-moving crowd from the dark, cool, low-ceilinged platform, he suddenly enters the immense concourse with its variety of heights and levels, its spaciousness, its acoustical properties, its diffused light, and the smooth texture of its floors and walls. Almost every sense is stimulated and flattered; even posture and gait are momentarily improved.

What Jackson is describing here sounds very much like the experience of constriction and release one feels passing through a dense forest and then stepping out into a broad clearing or meadow, the close, shadowy canopy of trees suddenly yielding to the soar of sky. Jackson writes that Grand Central, like many great architectural spaces, is among other things "an imitation of landscape"—of the various familiar forms of nature that precede architecture and have always supplied it with an especially rich trove of symbols. Owing to its scale, Grand Central is a particularly dramatic example of such an imitation, but the sequence of constriction and release we feel stepping out of a forest into a clearing is probably one of the most common spatial gestures, or tropes, in all architecture; even my little building contains it. It seems to me that spatial tropes of this kind—prospect and refuge is another—speak to us more deeply, more *physically*, than mere signs do, since our sense of their meaning depends on nothing more than the fact of our bodies and those forms of landscape with which everyone has had firsthand experience.

But if these examples seem too speculative, consider an even more elemental symbolism of space: vertical and horizontal, up and down, forward and back. Contrary to the teachings of Euclidean geometry, we don't really exist on an indifferent Cartesian grid, one where all spaces are alike and interchangeable, their coordinates given in the neutral terms of x, y, and z. Our bodies invest space with a very different set of coordinates, and these are no less real for being subjective. As Aristotle noted, up carries a very different connotation than down, front than back, inside than outside, vertical than horizontal. Vertical, for example, is more assertive than horizontal, associated as it is with standing up and the dominance such a posture affords, and though many of the meanings we attach to the vertical have grown more complicated than that (pride, hierarchy, aspiration, hubris, and so on), all are at bottom related to certain natural facts—specifically, to the upright stance of our species. Though something like verticality has been embroidered extensively by culture and history, its moral valence revised again and again (think of the fresh prestige Frank Lloyd Wright invested in the horizontal), its very meaningfulness—the basic terms on which an architect such as Wright could work his changes—is something given to us, not made. And it came into the world at the moment when our species first stood erect. Our bodies were making meaning out of the world long before our language had a chance to.

Our bodies are of course what get left out of a theory that treats architecture as a language, a system of signs. Such a theory can't explain the physical experience of two places as different as Grand Central Station and my little shack, because the quality of those experiences involves a tangle of mental *and* physical, cultural *and* biological elements that the theory can't account for, blinded as it is by old Western habits of regarding the mind and body as separate realms. Taking the side of the mind in the ancient dualism of mind and body, this theory can only explain that part of architecture that can be translated into words and pictures, published in magazines and debated at conferences. An architecture that ignores the body is certainly possible: the proof is all around us. But I doubt it will ever win our hearts.

It was to the body—to *my* body—that I owed the happy discovery that some of the reality I'd taken up a hammer to find was indeed still out there, and still available to me. I owed it to the body at rest, which had sensed in its shoulders the squeeze and release of the space in that room, but also to the body at work, sinking a chisel into the flesh of a Douglas fir, negotiating gravity in the raising of a roof beam. Not that I can ever hope to sort out all the different threads of sense and thought, body and mind, that have gone into the making of this experience (and this building), but then, that's precisely the point. It was only after my hands had woven a shelter from these slender leaves of cedar that my mind could grasp the poignancy of a shingle roof. Only after I'd raised onto its base a Douglas fir post fully as heavy as I am did I really understand the authority of a column.

To manhandle such a post into place, to join it to a beam that holds up a roof, is just the kind of work to remind you that, no matter how much cultural baggage can be piled onto something like a column (for as we've seen, it can signify republican virtue, South-

ern aristocracy, postmodern wit, and even deconstructivist violence), it is at bottom different from a word in a language. Though
perhaps a bit muffled by current architectural discourse, the architectural column still speaks to us of things as elemental as
standing up, of withstanding gravity, and of the trees that supported the roofs of our first homes on earth. It's not uninteresting
when Peter Eisenman takes such a column and suspends it from
the roof of a house so that it doesn't quite reach down to the
ground, but he is wrong to think my annoyance at the sight of it is
purely ideological, a matter of seeing a cherished cultural convention upset. Our regard for gravity is not just a question of taste.

It seems to me that as a metaphor for the process by which
architecture comes by its conventions, evolution is much more
useful than language. Certain architectural configurations (or patterns, to use Christopher Alexander's term) survive simply because
they have proven over time to be a good way to reconcile human
needs, the laws of nature, the facts of the human body, and the
materials at hand. Some of these patterns—load-bearing columns,
right angles, pitched roofs—appear almost everywhere we are, but
there are others that vary from place to place and from time to
time. Grand Central's spatial trope of constriction and release res-
onates most powerfully in a culture raised on a deeply forested
continent, in a place where the moment of coming into a clearing
has had a special urgency and savor. The important point is not
that these forms are necessarily universal or natural, but simply
that they are not arbitrary; they are the by-products of the things
and laws and processes of this world.

This is not a new idea, only a half-forgotten one, a fairly recent
casualty of the modern artist's cult of novelty. In architecture's first
treatise, Vitruvius describes a remarkably similar evolutionary process, and he was writing almost two thousand years before Darwin.
Vitruvius recounts the invention of the first building not as revelation but as a gradual process of trial and error involving many,

many builders, in which good ideas survived through imitation while bad ones fell by the wayside.

> And since [the first builders] were of an imitative and teachable na-
> ture, they would daily point out to each other the results of their
> building, boasting of the novelties in it; and thus, with their natural
> gifts sharpened by emulation, their standards improved daily. At first
> they set up forked stakes connected by twigs and covered these walls
> with mud . . . Finding that such roofs could not stand the rain dur-
> ing the storms of winter, they built them with peaks daubed with
> mud, the roofs sloping and projecting so as to carry off the rain
> water.

In Vitruvius' account good ideas are the ones most closely tuned to the nature of reality, something we only discover after the fact, by observing, and remembering, what works.

One of the advantages of using a metaphor of evolution like Vitruvius'—or, for that matter, Christopher Alexander's—to describe architecture is that it can take account of the tangled web of culture and nature we encounter in something like a building or in an architectural convention such as a column. It allows us to walk away from the cartoon opposition of nature and culture that has bewitched all builders of primitive huts, Peter Eisenman included. The human needs and the natural materials that go into the process of generating an architectural form are different from time to time and place to place; culture can enter into the process without rendering the whole thing arbitrary. It's worth remembering in this context that it was evolution that generated human culture—and language—in the first place, and that culture ever since has been working to modify evolution; notice the emphasis Vitruvius puts on talk—"boasting"—in the evolution of architecture.

A convention or pattern such as "windows on two sides of a room," which Alexander claims we value because it allows us to more readily read expressions off people's faces, might not work nearly so well in Japan, where shadowiness and reserve are prized more than psychological legibility. What this suggests is that the pattern is cultural without being in any way arbitrary, and that the process that generated it has a certain abiding logic. That logic, which is the same trial-and-error logic by which evolution proceeds, is the path out from the real things of this world to the forms of our architecture. It happens to be a path unavailable to our words; a writer or philosopher would be crazy *not* to envy it.

The mystery is, why would modern architecture ever want to turn away from this path, to trade such a distinction for a place in the common tub of images and information where I found it?

≡

That tub, this culture of ours so steeped in words and signs and images, poses a mortal challenge to architecture. For buildings aren't very well adapted to life in such an environment, one that puts a premium on mobility and ease of translation. Despite the best efforts of postmodern architects, buildings, unlike signs, don't travel well; they can't be digitized, and the good ones are dense with the kind of particularities and sense impressions that can't easily be summarized, much less sent over a wire or bounced off a satellite. About a memorable building we will often say "you had to be there," which is just another way of saying that the experience of the place, its presence, simply couldn't be translated into words and signs and information; the Here of it can't be communicated There.

You would think architects would cherish this about their work, if only because it makes architecture unique, a ballast amid the general weightlessness of an image culture. At least that's what I thought going in. As makers of real things that endure (things that get pointed to), didn't architects have it over the makers of words and images, those things that merely point, and that vanish as soon as the spotlight of our regard moves on? The work of building engaged them in a dialogue with the world, while the rest of us are lucky to add our two cents to the conversation of culture.

But apparently the prestige of that conversation is so great today that architecture, perhaps worried it was on its way to becoming dowdy and irrelevant, was desperate to find a place for itself nearer to the spotlit heart of our information society. So with the crucial help of Robert Venturi, who announced to his colleagues in *Learning from Las Vegas* that "the relevant revolution today is the current electronic one," architecture set about repackaging itself as a communications medium, playing down undigitizable space and experience—architecture's old brick-and-mortary Hereness—and playing up the literary or informational angle for all it was worth, until it seemed as though buildings were aspiring to the condition of television.

This has been a bad bargain, and not just for someone like me, who'd hoped by building to find a Here with which to counter the thrall of There in my life, but for architecture too. By allowing itself to become a kind of literary art, architecture might win itself a few more commissions from the Disney Company, but only at the price of giving up precisely what makes it different and valuable. Not that this troubles Robert Venturi. He has said he can't see much point in building grand public spaces anymore, now that television makes it possible to watch other people without leaving home.

As Venturi's comment suggests, the relationship between the information society and architecture may resemble a zero sum game. The culture of information is ultimately hostile to architecture, as it is to anything that can't be readily translated into its terms—to the whole of the undigitizable world, everything that the promoters of cyberspace like to refer to as RL (for "real life"). And yet notice how even these people are drawn to architectural and spatial metaphors, as if to acknowledge that, even now, architecture holds an enviable, inextinguishable claim on our sense of reality. Such terms as "cyberspace," "the electronic town hall," "cybershacks," "home pages," and "the information highway" belong to the great tradition of raiding architecture for its real-world palpableness— its *presence*—whenever someone's got something more abstract or ephemeral to sell. Once it was the philosophers, now it is the so-called digerati. The game, however, seems very much the same.

But architecture would do well to distrust this sort of flattery, because the cyberculture's interest in place is cynical and ulti-mately very slight. For what finally is the ultimate architectural ex-pression of the information culture we're being told is upon us? Try to picture *this* not-so-primitive hut: a roof, beneath which sits a man in a very comfortable, ergonomically correct chair, with a virtual reality helmet strapped around his head, an intravenous feeding hookup tethered to one arm, and some sort of toilet appa-ratus below. Think of him as Vitruvian man—the outstretched fig-ure in the circle in the square drawn by Da Vinci—updated for the twenty-first century. All that the information society really needs from architecture, apart from the comforting effect of its meta-phors, is a chair and a dry cybershack to house this body. Assum-ing, that is, the digerati don't succeed in their dream of completely downloading human consciousness into a computer, in which case the work left for architects, and the space left for these irre-deemable bodies of ours, will be skimpier still.

≡

I've built my own primitive hut according to a more old-fashioned blueprint; no doubt a deconstructivist would dismiss it as nos-talgic, or perhaps, considering its imperial prospects, danger-ously anthropocentric. But don't get the wrong idea: this is not Thoreau's crude shack in the woods that Joe and I have been build-ing. The blueprint calls not only for a telephone but a fax machine and a modem and a cubby for my computer; regarded from one

angle, mine is a kind of cybershack too, for this building and its oc-
cupant are going to be on-line, at least some of the time. (I am not
going in for the IV hookup, the VR helmet, or the toilet, however.)

From what I can tell so far, Charlie has designed me a building
that will provide a good counterweight to whatever information
and signs will be streaming into it (and my head) over that telephone wire—a credible enough Here with which to meet the
There on the line. He's given me plenty of reasons to gaze up from
the flickering screen, whether to check in on the view, scan the
bookshelves, or even contemplate the complicated underside of
my roof, which already exerts quite a presence in the room. It also
manages to keep out the rain, by the way: I checked this out at the
first opportunity, which came with a torrential thunderstorm a
couple of days after Joe and I had capped it. No roof is really done
until it has been tested by a storm; when this one came, I sprinted
out to the building as the summer rain slammed down, and nervously poked a flashlight beam up into the rafters, searching the
cedar shingles for telltale blotches or stains. There wasn't a one;
my roof was tight as a drum.

I sat for a while on the step waiting for the rain to subside,
watching it strafe the surface of the pond and fall from the eaves
in sheets. I think I enjoyed this rain as much as any I've been in,
listening to it tattoo the shingles overhead, producing an agreeable
clatter. Drop by drop it was testifying to the soundness of my roof,
reason enough to like it, but there was also the way the din seemed
to underscore the ceiling's beauty, the ear drawing the eye up into
the rafters, into that complicated weave of wood and work and
meaning that Charlie had dreamed up and Joe and I had actually
made.

I especially liked the way the lucid geometry of rafters and lath
set off the rough chiaroscuro of shingles, the one so very human in
its order and the other so reminiscent of tree bark and fish scales,
forest canopies and fields, of nature working in her best *e pluribus*

unum mode, fashioning something of beauty and consequence from simple slips of wood, leaves, blades of grass, and shadows. The juxtaposition of geometry and variousness set up a rhythm that was pleasing to the eye. It also brought out the character of the different woods, the long, legible grain of the fir throwing into relief the furriness of cedar, and this along with the visual rhythm gave my roof an almost emphatic Hereness.

Present it most certainly seemed to be. And yet at the same time the ceiling seemed to *re-present* too, offering up its allusions to boat hulls and leaf canopies, tree houses and classical dentils, a web of allusion fully as complex and layered as the weave of its wood and workmanship. So which was it, Here or There? Not either/or, I decided, but *both*: Here *and* There, shelter and symbol, nature and culture at once. And then it occurred to me, as I gazed out at the view down toward my arbor, just then draped in the velvety purple vestments of a *clematis jackmanii*, that a building was probably less like a text than a garden. For it is the garden that manages, in a way that few things in this life do, to celebrate the here and now (with its full complement of sensory satisfactions) while at the same time summoning the there and then by means of its symbolism. The garden's mode is not metaphor exactly—one thing for another—but something else: one thing *and* another. Unlike a painting of a landscape, say, or a poem about nature, behind which stands nothing but pigment or marks on a page, the garden offers us an experience whose power does not depend on codes or conventions or even the suspension of disbelief, though all those things are at work here too, making the experience that much richer.

So, I guess you could say I liked my roof well enough. Already it had proven itself capable not only of keeping the rain off my head, which you'll have to take my word for, but also of housing the far-flung speculations of its builder, whose soundness you can judge for yourself. Thoreau regretted he hadn't put a somewhat bigger and higher roof over his head at Walden, since "you want room for your thoughts to get into sailing trim and run a course or two before they make their port . . . Our sentences [want] room to unfold." My roof, my place, promised at least that much: to offer a decent habitation for my thoughts. But something more too, something specific to my life and perhaps my times as well. Out there in this new room of mine, dryly enjoying the summer rain with its fine tang of ozone, it seemed just the place to sit and compose a word or two on behalf of the sights and sounds and senses of this, our still undigitized world.

Windows

By the time Joe and I headed into the second winter of construction, our work together, even though it amounted to something less than one day a week, had acquired its own particular rhythms and textures and talk. Joe reveled in playing the role of mentor to my eager if still-somewhat maladroit apprentice, except for the occasional period of sulking, when he would temporarily revert to sullen clock-puncher. These episodes were invariably occasioned by a suggestion from me that we should perhaps consult the blueprints before undertaking framing a window opening or hanging a door. "You mean the funny papers," Joe'd grumble. "Well, you're the boss," he'd shrug, egging me to take control, or sides; I never was quite sure which. But in time such episodes became more rare, for as my own confidence as a carpenter grew, I was less inclined to regard Charlie's drawings as revealed truth, much to Joe's satisfaction.

Working outside in the brief, chill days of December had a way of hurrying this process along. Architectural plans look different in the cold, especially when you're rocking stiffly from boot to boot on top of fossilized mud, dispatching neural messages to toes and fingertips that go unheeded, and struggling to interpret lines on a drawing that only seem more ambiguous the harder you stare at them. *Joe, can you see any framing to hold up that window? Nope, not a stick. Looks like he wants us to levitate this one.* Under such circumstances the solidarity of carpenters is bound to intensify. After a while you can't look at the blueprints—which by now have had their pristine geometries smudged by a parade of muddy thumbs—without thinking about the comfortable office in which they were drawn, the central heating and scrubbed fingernails and steaming pots of coffee. Such images had a way of magnifying any lapses in the architect's renderings into affronts, any peculiarities of design into definitive proof of the woolly-headedness of the professional classes that do their work indoors. A class to which, it was true, I'd be returning myself first thing Monday, but for the time being my allegiance was to the double-gloved, triple-socked, shivering and quick-to-get-pissed-off outdoor crew.

It was an allegiance I found myself compelled to declare late one December afternoon, to Joe's unbounded delight. He had casually called my attention to a notation on the drawings that specified pine, of all things, for the piece of wood that framed the recessed rock window on the building's north exterior wall. It never occurred to me this might be some sort of a test, but I passed it just the same. "Fuck that," I said, surprising myself almost as much as Joe. Pine was a dumb idea on several counts: the shady north side promised to be perpetually damp (pine has no rot resistance to speak of) and every single other piece of exposed exterior lumber—from the roofing shingles to the trim—was cedar, of which we happened to have several beautiful lengths left. "We're going to use one-inch clear cedar there, I don't care what the drawings say," I announced, and Joe erupted. "*Yes!* You've finally got it!" he shouted, launching into a gleeful little end-zone dance in the snow. "Mike, I have been waiting an entire year to hear you speak those fine words. Charlie's down . . . he's *out!*"

But sometimes Joe could take the Professor Higgins act a little too far. Probably because I'd proven such a willing pupil in matters of carpentry, Joe eventually began to think there might be other areas in which I stood to benefit from his instruction, and I soon found myself on the receiving end of lengthy lectures about child rearing, television, economics, and politics. I wouldn't have minded this too much, conversation being one of carpentry's best perks, except that Joe had a habit of stopping whatever job he was doing in advance of making a point and then forestalling its resumption until I had more or less conceded the wisdom of his argument. When we got to gun control—and sooner or later we always got to gun control—work all but ground to a halt.

I knew politics were on tap whenever Joe'd pop his hammer into its holster, rear back on his heels, and then lean forward punching the air with his index finger. Power tools silenced, the woods would ring with his rhetorical question: "Mike, do you want to know what's really wrong with this country?" Whether the abomination of the day was crime or immigration or free trade or the varieties of idiocy regnant in Washington and Hartford, the monologue would somehow or other and often quite ingeniously wend its way back to the mother subject of gun control. The precise route we would travel from here to there I never could quite reconstruct—the transitions could be dazzling—but get there we would, and before it was all over I'd be treated to a soaring peroration from some Second Amendment deity whom he'd then challenge me to identify.

" 'Before a standing army can rule, the people must be disarmed; as they are in almost every kingdom of Europe. The supreme power in America cannot enforce unjust laws by the sword; because the whole body of the people are armed, and constitute a force superior to any bands of regular troops . . .' "

"Jefferson?"

"Guess again."

"Tom Paine?"

"*Wrong*. Noah Webster, 1787. I thought you said you went to college."

The jurisprudence of the Second Amendment was Joe's specialty; no other amendment (and least of all numbers four, five, and eight) elicited the same fervent devotion. (Indeed, he believed that the solution to the crime problem involved crueler and more unusual punishment.) Joe was not himself a serious hunter, but he collected guns and knew an astounding amount about their history and technology, their lore and care and proper handling. Any time we heard the report of a hunter's rifle, he would stop to announce the caliber of the gun in question and then proceed to enumerate its salient virtues and limitations. Joe was convinced that if I would only learn more about guns, I would not be so quick to endorse ignorant measures like the Brady Bill and the assault weapons ban—which anyone with any sense at all and about $50 worth of mail-order parts could *easily* circumvent, and which—was I aware of this?—specifically exempted assault weapons manufactured by the Israelis. Joe left me with back issues of *Shotgun News* and all manner of NRA propaganda; once he presented me with a bullet of some advanced design that allowed it to travel just under the speed of sound so as not to make a sonic boom.

Like many people who regard gun control as the preeminent threat to our liberties, Joe's politics occasionally shaded off into areas you really didn't care to visit, the kind of places where the fantasies of Oliver Stone and the militia movement begin to fuzz together. I'm not entirely sure, though, whether it was the arrayed forces of conspiracy or stupidity that Joe deemed the greater threat; nor was I sure which offered safer conversational ground. Joe and I could just about agree on the folly of free trade or the perfidy of the Bureau of Alcohol, Tobacco, and Firearms, but when he'd start in on his theories of evolution—how people are growing progressively more stupid because technology and the welfare state are interfering with the proper functioning of natural selection—I worked hard to steer him back to the relative safety of the Bill of Rights or, best and most benign of all, the perversity of architects.

On this last theme, Joe and I had lately found a broad stretch of common ground. We had coined a term that we hauled out regularly to damn anything in Charlie's plans that in our estimation defied practicality or common sense: "Eight-one." It was sort of like the cop's "ten-four," or the short-order cook's "eighty-six." The pine window trim was an eight-one, so was its thin-air framing; in fact, the windows taken as a whole were one great big eight-one, since they were designed, as windows in the real world very seldom are, to open inward rather than out. This and a few other details about their design meant the windows could not be ordered out of a catalog but would have to be custom-made at considerable expense. "Custom" would be a very generous translation of our "eight-one."

Why "eight-one"? The term derived from the 8'1" height Charlie had specified for the walls in the main part of the building, a dimension calculated to offend every fiber in the body of any self-respecting carpenter. Lumber comes in standard even-numbered lengths; two-by-fours are either eight, ten, or twelve feet long, and plywood sheets come four by eight. Indeed, eight feet is virtually the common denominator of American construction, going all the way back to the standard dimension of a bay in Colonial houses and barns; ever since, the number eight has been one of the more prestigious integers in carpentry. In order to make all the 8'1" two-by-fours and lengths of plywood we would need to complete our walls and fin walls, a tremendous amount of wood would have to be wasted, not to mention sawing time, and, to a carpenter, waste is one of the forms poor craftsmanship takes. Whatever the architectural logic that dictated designing a wall one inch off of such a canonical dimension, to a carpenter it represented sheer perversity, a slap in the face of tradition, common sense, and frugality. Indeed you could argue—and believe me, Joe did—Charlie's eight-one summed up everything that was wrong with the practice of architecture in America today.

I remembered once reading a story in *Fine Homebuilding*, the magazine for carpenters and serious do-it-your-selfers, about a contractor who had grown so sick of performing what he regarded as needlessly "custom" work for architects that, when the time came to design a house for himself, he made sure that every last piece of wood in it would be a standard dimension, the overwhelming majority of them eight feet. The ceilings were eight feet, the floor plan of every story and room was a multiple of eight, and all the windows and door openings were a simple fraction of eight. This fellow bragged of the fact that not only had he designed his house without an architect, but he had been able to more or less frame it without using a saw. But what made him proudest of all was that not a single piece of framing lumber had gone to waste.

"And have you actually *seen* this house?" Charlie demanded to know when I told him the story. He was in town checking on another job, and had stopped by at the end of the day to go over a couple of problems that had cropped up in the plans. Joe and I'd been giving him a hard time about the eight-one walls and the in-swinging windows, the full scope of whose difficulty—their radical customness—having just sailed into view. The day before, I'd taken Charlie's drawings to a millworker who'd informed me that not only would the windows as drawn cost several thousand dollars to fabricate, but that he couldn't guarantee they wouldn't leak. I intended to get around to this before Charlie left town.

"Because my guess is that this Mister Eight-Oh of yours lives in one god-awful box. Oh sure, nobody actually *needs* an architect, if all you want is shelter, a dry box to work in. But you wanted something more."

True enough, but surely architecture doesn't require eight-one walls.

"Actually, I would argue that sometimes it does." Charlie was clearly ready for us this time, and in no mood to let a pair of cranky weekend carpenters trash his profession. Charlie had come from a meeting on a new job he'd landed nearby; he was wearing his country-client attire, a graph-paper-checked shirt, chinos, and a sweater vest that together managed deftly to say to the client: informal yet billable. (Thankfully Charlie had taken my own job off the clock several months earlier, after I'd made some noises about the magnitude of the initial design fees.)

Charlie reached into the rank of pens lining his breast pocket. Taking a black Expresso Bold to our smeary copy of the blueprint, he proceeded to demonstrate how he'd arrived at the eight-one dimension, a complex puzzle revolving around the need to keep both the height of the door and the building's distance from the ground at a bare minimum. "One inch less in that wall and the doorjamb on the landing would be grazing your head. I suppose I could have raised the lower floor an inch, like so, but then the front elevation starts to float—not good. And when I start *adding* inches to the height of the wall, entering the building isn't nearly so nice—you lose that neat transition from low, tight doorway into big space. *Way* too ordinary." It was reassuring to know that eight-one hadn't been an oversight. But I didn't buy that raising the floor one inch would have ruined the elevation.

"And by the way," Charlie continued, hoisting his bushy eyebrows over an expression of mock injury, "the term 'custom' is a much friendlier way to describe what I do than this rude 'eight-one' business."

Charlie's disdain for the "way too ordinary" reminded me of a definition Le Corbusier had once proposed for architecture. Architecture, Le Corbusier had declared, is when the windows are either too big or too small, but never the "right" size. For when the window is the right size, the building is . . . just a building. Viewed from one perspective, Le Corbusier's dictum is as succinct a confession of artistic arrogance as you could ask for, implying as it did that originality, if not eccentricity, was an end in itself. Architecture as the wrong-size window is precisely what had sent Mister Eight-Oh around the bend—and what made his radically stock response seem at least partly sane.

And yet, as Charlie was suggesting, where would you rather spend the afternoon? In the Villa Savoye, or Mr. Eight-Oh's House of the Standard Dimensions? "Any building that's trying not just to give shelter but to move us—to raise our spirits—is bound to break with our expectations in all sorts of ways," Charlie said. "Sometimes you have to italicize a door or a window in order to make people see it freshly, and that might very well mean making it 'too big' or 'too small.' The fact is, your Mister Eight-Oh may have saved himself some trouble and some dough, but he's missing out on the soul of a good building."

Joe now tried to reel the conversation back down to earth, where he hoped to pick up some needed information and then with any luck call it a day.

"I hear what you're saying about seeing things fresh, Charlie. But there are a couple things in these drawings of yours we can't see *at all*—like the framing for this little rock window here. Sometimes Mike forgets to rub the lemon juice on these things and we can't read the invisible ink."

"Hey. Mike here knows all about invisible ink—that's what he signs his checks with. But I hear you. I'll fax you an S-K on that tomorrow." "S-K" is architect talk for "sketch," which seems a rather dubious abbreviation when you realize it actually takes longer to pronounce than the word it purports to crop. Evidently

a certain amount of opaque insider talk is a professional imperative; indeed, without an inside and an outside you probably don't
have a profession.

All this backing and forthing was really just a warm-up for the
talk we needed to have about the windows, the biggest eight-one of
them all. All told there were eight of them, in five distinct types
(the two big in-swinging awnings at either end of the building; one
single-sash casement that swung out on the north wall overlooking
the rock; one double-sash in-swinging French casement on the
south wall, and then the two fixed and two operable windows in
the peak)—all in a building not a whole lot bigger than a minivan.
According to the lumberyard, only one of them—the out-swinging
casement that would overlook the rock—was a stock item; the rest
were as custom as custom gets. I told Charlie that the first millworker I'd taken them to, a giant, dour Swede named Tude Tanguay, had taken one look at the drawing of the awning window and
pronounced it worthless. Tude guessed it *might* be possible to
design an in-swinging window that didn't let in the rain, but he
was sure of one thing: This wasn't that. "Architects," Tude had
growled, adopting the tone of voice other people reserve for the
words "termites" or "telemarketers." "Fellow who drew this doesn't
even show a drip edge," he pointed out, pushing the blueprint
aside. "Get me a better detail, then we'll talk."

Charlie acknowledged he needed to come up with a system to prevent water from seeping under the sash and promised to get
me a sketch right away. Very gingerly, I asked him if maybe we
shouldn't reconsider the whole approach. Couldn't we find stock
windows that would give us at least part of what we wanted, for a lot
less money and with some assurance they wouldn't leak? But Charlie
felt strongly that the windows were the wrong place to compromise.

"These in-swinging awning windows are absolutely key to the
scheme. Remember, the whole idea here was to make the end
walls vanish in summer—to turn your building into a porch. I don't
know of any better way to do that than with these windows." He

proceeded to tick off each of the stock solutions he'd considered—double-hungs, casements, and ordinary awnings—and explain why none would give us the effect we were looking for. In every case, the open window would leave a frame of mullions or visible sash instead of landscape wall to wall.

"These windows are your building's face, Mike, your face and your frame. They set up the whole relationship between inside and outside, between the guy sitting in that chair and the landscape. To use stock windows here would be like buying those cheapo reading glasses they sell off the rack at Woolworth's. Maybe they do the job, I don't know. But you can't say it's the same thing as having your own prescription. That's what these are: prescription windows."

Joe was rolling his eyes. As he listened to Charlie talk, he'd been peeling off one layer of outerwear after another, getting ready to head home, and he'd stopped at a frayed black T-shirt with purple lettering across the chest that said, "What part of NO don't you understand?" This was right up there in Joe's collection of heavy-metal hostile-wear with his UZI DOES IT T-shirt. I told Charlie to fax me a detail for the windows. We'd see if we couldn't figure out a way to make them work.

≡

The problem with in-swinging windows, the reason you don't often see them in this world, is best understood by comparing two drawings:

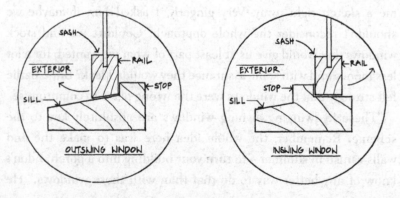

In a conventional out-swinging window (the one on the left), the stop against which the sash rests also serves as a weather barrier, effectively returning any water that seeps under the bottom edge of the sash back down the sill and away from the building. (The same holds true in a common double-hung window.) But when the window sash opens inward, which it can't do unless the stop is to its outside, a certain amount of the rainwater that runs down the pane will find its way between the sash and the stop, and from there into the room. This is by no means a simple problem to solve. There is a very good reason for most windows to open outward; given the predictable behavior of water when presented with opportunities to infiltrate a building, a sash that swings out is the easiest and most natural solution, the fenestral equivalent of a pitched roof. Which is not to say the convention cannot be successfully defied, only that doing so will demand a more elaborate technology, and perhaps a greater degree of imagination on the part of its designer. It would help, for example, for the designer of such a window to be able to think like water, in the words of an old gardener I once knew.

When a few days later I received Charlie's window detail, I wasn't at all sure he had solved the problem. Basically what Charlie had come up with was a rubber gasket to close off the gap between sash and stop, as follows:

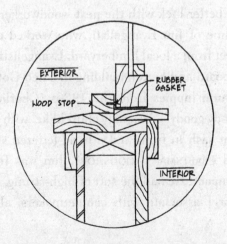

Thinking like water, I could easily imagine working my way down as far as that gasket, where it seemed to me I would be apt to linger and eventually do some damage to the surrounding wood, or maybe freeze and thaw enough times to crack the rubber gasket and then find my way indoors.

But what did I know? I wasn't an architect, and I was only maybe half a carpenter, if that.

So I took Charlie's detail back to Tude Tanguay, whom I found up in the woods behind his shop, slicing oak trunks into logs with a chain saw so easily they might have been baguettes. It was a threatening December morning, and the chill in the air was raw, arthritic. The big man had a black watch cap pulled down over his ears, and his Honest Abe half-beard was fringed with ice crystals. I felt like I was delivering a piece of unsolicited mail to Paul Bunyan. The detail was useless, Tude declared after a cursory glance at the paper, and for more or less the reasons I'd suspected. Yet whatever satisfaction I might have taken in being right was overshadowed by the grim realization that my architect seemed to know rather less about designing a weatherproof window than I did: a quite serious problem. I asked Tude if he had any suggestions.

"Not off the top," he said, gunning his chain saw. "Let me think on it, get back to you."

Sure.

I had much better luck with the next woodworker I tried, a fellow by the name of Jim Evangelisti, who worked out of a shop across the street from a local lumberyard. Evangelisti's shop was in a tall-gabled, board-and-batten building in a neo-Gothic style I associate with rural hippies from the 1970s (Charlie would have called it a "woody goody")—vaguely churchlike, with a soaring wall of divided-light sash in front and a hand-lettered sign above the door that said CRAFTSMAN WOODSHOPS. Jim was fortyish, sandy haired and compact. He had the sort of high-strung, slightly squirrelly demeanor I associate with cabinetmakers, along with the usual complement of smashed-up fingers. It hurt mine just to look at them.

It was a couple of weeks before Christmas when I dropped by with my drawings, and Jim was doing some pro bono work on the Christmas display for Main Street, drilling holes for lights in a plywood Santa, a mentholated cigarette clamped between his teeth. I didn't get the feeling there was a backlog of work in-house; Jim showed considerably more interest in my project than Tude Tanguay had, though he was precisely as flattering as Tude had been about Charlie's window detail.

"Well *this* isn't going to do us any good," he said, flicking his fingers loudly against Charlie's page. "You'll have standing water on that stop, and he's put his gasket way too far down—you can't have water collecting *there*. You should also know right now I don't make sash the way he's showing it, with stops to hold the panes. I mount the glass with putty, same way it's been done in New England for three hundred years at least." Then he lit up another Kool and waved Charlie's drawing at me. "You know what I call these?"

"Let me guess . . ."

"*Cartoons.*"

But when I asked him if he had a better idea, he actually did . . . sort of. Jim said that Greene and Greene, the California architects who specialized in bungalow-style houses around the turn of the century, had built the only successful in-swinging casement windows he had ever seen. It seems that Jim had worked on the renovation of a Greene and Greene house in Berkeley after he got out of college in the mid-seventies. He couldn't remember exactly how the casements worked, only that they'd had an unusually steep sill and some sort of drip edge. "But most of the Greene and Greene drawings are at Columbia University. Maybe you could find a detail."

We agreed I would look for one, while Jim worked up a price. But I hesitated. My confidence in Charlie's window scheme was dwindling, and I was seriously considering bailing out on it, sacrificing what might well be a set of brilliant ideas to the legitimate demands of practicality. Though really, how brilliant was any architectural idea that so blithely defied the facts, the exigencies of construction and weather, which is to say the world we live in? It seemed to me Charlie had really dropped the ball on this one, that he had designed me the equivalent of a modernist leaky roof, an interesting but unworkable conceit. I was going to wind up like one of those quietly fuming clients of modern architecture who, when they dare complain to the master about the back-breaking chair or the drip on their heads, are forced to endure one of those delightful, one-eye-on-the-biographer quips about buckets and genius. ("This is what happens," sighed one of Frank Lloyd Wright's clients, resigned to her leaking house, "when you leave a work of art out in the rain.") The willingness of people in this century to suffer on behalf of art (and someone *else's* art, at that) may have been a precondition for the rise of modern architecture, but it wasn't something I wanted any part of.

And yet . . . there was the promise of those prescription windows. Every window is an interpretation of a landscape, and the variety and inventiveness of Charlie's fenestration, so specific to the site and circumstance (so custom, in the very best sense), was one of the most exciting parts of his design. What a sweet idea, to turn the writing house into a porch for the summer; Charlie's metaphor of putting the top down on the convertible had stayed with me. Windows that opened in would also, I imagined, admit the landscape to the building, usher in that cascade of space, of chi, that had attracted me to the site in the first place. And I particularly liked the idea of the windows on each of the thick walls with their extreme close-up views: the hump of gray-green rock on my right and the tangled, fragrant, light-filtering vine on the south side, both shelved right there alongside my books.

So, sure, I was taken with the romance of these windows—this novel pair of glasses, eight lenses custom-ground. And yet every whisper of that tiny, hissing, deflationary word—"leak"—put my head in a mind to overrule my heart's desire.

I couldn't decide the question one way or the other for more than a minute at a time, so I figured I might as well pay a visit to Avery Library at Columbia, check out Jim's tip. If I found a Greene and Greene window detail that looked like it might work, fine; if not, I would insist that Charlie redesign the windows. Over the phone, the librarian at the archive confirmed that they did indeed have a sizable collection of original Greene and Greene drawings—several thousand of them, in fact. I couldn't decide whether this was good news or not; I certainly wasn't about to spend a week chasing down the drip edge Charlie had dropped. The librarian didn't know anything about window details per se (why would she?), but said that all the drawings had recently been put on a CD-ROM, which meant I could flip through them pretty quickly. I made an appointment for the following morning.

The resolution of the images on the CD-ROM was too poor for me to discern whether any given window opened in or out, but it allowed me to narrow my search to a series of houses with promising-looking casements. The librarian pulled my selections from the file drawers, spreading the delicate buff pencil drawings on a table while reciting the archive's rules: no photocopying, no tracing, no ballpoint pens or ink markers on the table. Great. The last best hope for my windows, if not for the integrity of my building's design, rested on my skill as a freehand draftsman, which was exactly nil.

I washed my hands and started going through the drawings. Most of the houses pictured were elaborately timbered bungalows with a great many shallow gables piled one on top of the other in a manner reminiscent of Japanese architecture. You could see why a cabinetmaker who called his business the Craftsman Woodshops would respond to this work: the Greenes' designs owed a lot to the Arts and Crafts movement, sharing its emphasis on traditional craftsmanship in wood. With their exposed structures and hand-worked finishes, many of the houses look like celebrations of the very possibilities of wood and the art of joinery; they exhibited in their design and finishes a kind of transparency to the craftsmanship that made them. Coming at a time when such craftsmanship was under attack from the factory system, such an aesthetic had a strong moral cast, made a last-gasp protest against the machine age and an assertion of the dignity of work. It is a message that still seems to speak to many carpenters today (and not only to them).

By the end of the morning, I had found what I was looking for: an ingenious construction detail for an in-swinging casement window on a house in Pasadena. I kept going, and began to find variations on the same idea over and over again, in one house after another. The window must have worked, I reasoned, or else the Greenes would have tried some radically different tack or given up on the in-swing altogether. So I copied the window detail into my notebook as carefully as I could, checking it once and then again to make sure I'd left nothing important out (assuming of course that I knew what important looked like).

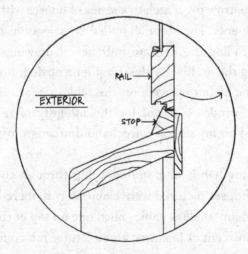

To my inexpert eye it seemed a fine solution, economical in the best sense. The bottom frame of the sash, or rail, doubled as a drip edge; by designing the rail to overhang the stop, the designer ensured that any water coming down along its face would fall onto the sill rather than the stop. And the curved profile of the stop itself eliminated any surface on which water might linger. At first I didn't understand the purpose of the groove routed into the underside of the sash, but when I brought the drawing to Jim the following Saturday, he grasped its significance immediately.

"Capillary action. Water wants to migrate along the underside of a surface, so it'll work its way back to that gap there unless something is put in its way. That's what the groove's for: Water will collect in it until the bead gets heavy enough to break the surface tension. Then it'll drop onto the sloping side of that stop and down to the sill and away." Here was a case of thinking like water at the Ph.D. level.

Jim felt the detail was definitely workable, though he'd need to adapt it some. For one thing, Connecticut gets a lot more rainfall than California does; for another, my windows would be made of painted pine rather than unfinished redwood (far too heavy for sash this size, never mind the expense), and he worried about the ability of such a slender pine stop to withstand the weight of sash banging against it. But he had some ideas. Jim gave me his price, which seemed fair in view of the complexities. It was, however, somewhat more than I could afford. Jim suggested I could shave several hundred dollars off of the total if I was willing to make the four little peak windows myself, a job he assured me was fairly straightforward. So we pulled these items out of the deal and shook hands on it.

≡

Jim had said it would be okay with him if I wanted to watch him build the windows, so early on a Monday morning I came by his shop. On a pallet by the front door stood a short stack of fresh, rough-sawn white pine planks of various lengths, knot-free and covered in a soft blond down. Nothing about this wood made you think "window"; it could not have been more opaque or inert. And yet what Jim proposed to do before the morning was over was transform this stack of lumber into intricate skeletons of finished white pine, the airy frames of six divided-light windows. The singleness of "stock"—what Jim called the raw pine—would be translated into that rich, antique, and multifarious vocabulary English offers for the parts of a window: sashes and stiles, muntins and mullions, sills and jambs and rails and casings and lights.

Jim's shop consisted of two large rooms divided by wooden racks stacked with handsome slabs of unfinished oak, cherry, mahogany, maple, and pine. Both spaces were crowded with doors, windows, cabinets, and countertops arrested in various stages of fabrication, and the whole place looked as though a blizzard had recently passed through, coating everything in several inches of fresh, fragrant sawdust, Jim included. The back room held two large, low tables where Jim did his layouts and glue-ups. Up front were a half-dozen machine tools spread out around the room in a rough approximation of an assembly line, separate stations each for the planer, shaper, table saw, tenoner, mortiser, and drill punch. It seemed like an awful lot of machinery for a woodworker as devoted to tradition as Jim professed to be.

"They've improved on the chisel some," Jim said as he set to work, bunching the sleeves of his sweatshirt at the elbows, "but the mortise joint is still the best we know how to make." In this Jim's thinking was in keeping with the Arts and Crafts movement for which he obviously felt a kinship. Gustav Stickley, the turn-of-the-century furniture maker who promoted Arts and Crafts ideas in America, had objected not to the machine as such but to the uses to which it was being put, including mass production and the devaluing of craftsmanship. "When rightly used," Stickley had written in *The Craftsman*, the influential magazine he began publishing in 1900, "the machine is simply a tool in the hand of a skilled worker."

In Jim's hands, the machine was a howling and slightly terrifying agent of transformation. Working with a swiftness that went some distance toward explaining the condition of his fingers, Jim escorted each rough plank from one station to the next, guiding the pine along on a journey of ever-increasing refinement and specificity. First he would select a piece of stock from the pile by the door and feed it through the planer, a steel sandwich of spinning blades that peeled a thin, even layer from both sides of the wood at once, leaving it smooth and plumb. Now Jim would lay the piece down against a full-scale diagram of the window he'd drawn on a masonite board, decide on its role (muntin, stile, rail, etc.) then mark it for width and length and cut it on the table saw. Next the stock would enter the snout of the shaper, from which it emerged looking like a piece of finished molding, its square corners having acquired the curved profile of a coping or fillet, ogee or reverse ogee, depending on the bit used. Shouting over the scream of the machine, Jim said that shaper bits cost upward of a thousand dollars apiece, so it was tough luck if I didn't like the one he owned. My windows received the same austere profile you see all over New England, their crossbars, or muntins, narrowing down from glass pane to nosing in three quick curving steps, each about half the size of the one preceding. Not too finicky, but not too plain either; I liked it fine.

From here on, the destiny of the various pieces of stock diverged, as some were designated tenons and others mortises, male or female depending on how they would ultimately fit into the window frame. The muntin bars that would hold the panes of glass in place would all be tenoned into the stiles and rails for maximum strength; each muntin passed through a tenoning machine that whittled its ends down to a narrow rectangular tongue of wood. The beefier members that would receive the muntin bars went instead to the mortiser, a modified drill press that cut perfectly matched notches using a spinning bit in combination with a chisel. Every one of these machines looked and sounded hungry for fingertips.

Once all the pieces had been cut and shaped, Jim spread them out on his worktable and began fitting them together, like a puzzle. With a gentle tap of his wooden mallet, the tenons snapped smartly into their notches, the molding designs neatly turning the corners and matching up, concave fillets meeting fillets, convex copings meeting copings. The machine tolerances were so exact that, except for the largest sash, whole frames virtually squared themselves. Satisfied with the fit, Jim would take the frames apart, spread glue over tenons and into notches, and then reassemble them. After checking for square, he'd clamp the frames end to end and put them aside to dry. In a day or two, he'd send the frames out to the man who did his glazing. "There's a knack to working the putty just right," he explained when I asked why he subbed out this particular step. "Glazing's an old-timer's game."

Once the frames were assembled, I studied Jim's drip edge detail. It looked like this:

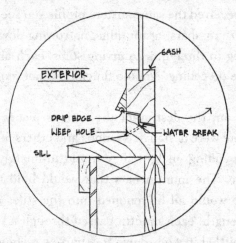

It was ingenious, if not quite as economical as the Greene and Greene detail on which it was based. Like theirs, the bottom edge of my sash extended well out over the stop, in order to conduct water away from the window, and it had a groove routed along its underside to thwart any capillary action. But below, the design diverged from its model, since Jim had decided he couldn't taper the stop, as the Greenes had done, to minimize its surface area. Pine wouldn't have been strong enough, for one thing. But the more serious problem, and the one I never saw coming, was that in an awning window (as opposed to a casement like the Greenes') when the projecting drip edge swung inward, it would follow a slight downward arc that would actually collide with any stop that wasn't either set well beneath it or angled the *wrong* way—that is, toward the building's interior, rather than away. (You had to think like wood as well as water in this business.) Jim's solution was inspired: He angled the stop toward the building so that the drip edge would clear it coming in. Then he routed a second groove along its surface to collect any water seeping under the sash, which would then flow out through a series of weep holes drilled through the stop. Basically, Jim had provided a second line of defense.

I congratulated him on the design, a critical detail of my building that no one except perhaps another carpenter would probably ever notice. Jim was unexpectedly cranky about it. "I'm not going to start complaining yet, but I've got two extra days in this job already, just thinking. Architects get a lot of money to come up with this kind of detail." Maybe, but it seemed to me that this is precisely the place where, nowadays at least, architecture stops, where it comes down either to finding a craftsman like Jim Evangelisti or a bucket.

Except for the tapping of the wooden mallet, the final assembly was mercifully quiet, and Jim talked a little about the path that had brought him to the Craftsman Woodshops, which turned out not to be so far from where he started. Jim's family had owned the lumberyard across the street, so he'd always been around wood and carpenters as a kid, but it wasn't until he went away to college, in Vermont, that he got serious about woodworking. One of his professors at

Godard was building an authentic timber frame house, cutting his own wood off the site, milling it by hand, and framing the structure solely with hand tools—no electricity allowed. It was the seventies, remember, and Vermont was teeming with back-to-the-land types who (not unlike members of the Arts and Crafts movement) made a moral and political virtue of traditional craftsmanship and self-reliance.

After college Jim moved out to California, where he heard about the restoration of a Greene and Greene house in Berkeley. "I saw right away that the architect in charge didn't have a clue," Jim said. "I mean, he was *butt*-jointing everything for chrissake! Didn't know the first thing about the joinery in that house. I practically had to force them to let me work on it." As I listened to Jim describe the months he spent on the job—replacing a porch railing and restoring an ornate footbridge that he still had a dog-eared drawing of—I could see that the job had been a high point for him, and a formative experience. He'd found his calling. That, and his lifelong bête noire: the well-paid and ignorant architects he always seemed to end up bailing out.

And yet, Jim's architect-bashing aside, it seemed to me he and Charlie had important things in common. Not least was their deep appreciation for the American vernacular and the indigenous architecture that had drawn on it so fruitfully before modernism turned everybody's attention back to Europe. Charlie and Jim were both children of the seventies, their approach toward building having been shaped by an odd confluence of currents that was at the time helping to return American architecture to American sources. One of these currents was of course postmodernism, which by the mid-seventies had sparked a revival of interest in the American shingle style, a homegrown domestic architecture with deep vernacular roots. Also gathering momentum during the seventies was the push for historic preservation. And then, coming from an entirely different quarter, there was the back-to-the-land movement, which had its own reasons to revive vernacular building styles and methods, such as timber framing; it also happened to share many of the values of the Arts and Crafts movement. (You remember the crafts.) Though it seldom finds its way into the architectural histories, American hippie architecture of the 1970s played an important role, chipping away at modernist ideas from below while more academic postmodernists attacked them head on. So while Jim was lending a hand to the revival of timber framing in Vermont, Charlie was studying at UCLA under Charles Moore, the postmodernist with perhaps the deepest feeling for the American vernacular.

In fact it wouldn't be too much to say that Jim and Charlie, having started out from two such different places, had been working their way toward the very sort of neotraditional window coming together on this worktable at the Craftsman Woodshops. For the divided-light window, along with timber framing, pitched roofs, wooden shingles, and a great many other vernacular elements, was one of the casualties of modernism that architects like Charlie and craftsmen like Jim have both done their parts to revive. Here in microcosm was that collaboration, between the postmodern temper and the craftsman ideal—the "neo" and the "traditional." Not that the collaboration was an easy or even a friendly one. The architect, being a modern artist, was not content merely to revive an idiom but insisted on giving it a fresh turn (the too-big window, the inswinging sash), his novelty forcing the craftsman back on his wits (and his memory of forgotten solutions, such as the Greenes' drip edge) to make it all work. Or to bail him out, depending on your point of view.

≡

Of all the revivals of the postmodern period, perhaps the most surprising is the divided-light window. The pitched roof, after all, could justify its return strictly on utilitarian grounds: a case can be made that a gable was simply the best way to keep the weather out of a house. But the muntin bars dividing a window into small panes of glass can make no such claim for themselves. Indeed, from a purely technological standpoint, they have been obsolete in all but the very largest windows since the invention of rolled sheet glass near the end of the eighteenth century. It isn't until the modern period, however, that they disappeared completely, only to be brought back again in the last few years—thanks (once again) to Robert Venturi, who put a gigantic, divided-light window on the façade of his mother's house. (Actually it's a sliding glass door bisected by a thick horizontal muntin bar.) The story of the fall and rise of the humble muntin, which I started looking into after my time in Jim Evangelisti's shop, turns out to shed some light not only on how my own particular windows came to be, but on the whole history of the idea of transparency in the West, which is itself a kind of sub-history of our changing attitudes toward nature, objectivity, and the notion of perspective—a person's and a building's both.

Muntins were originally invented as a way to gang together numerous small panes of glass when that was the only kind there was. Before the development of sheet glass, a windowpane was made by blowing a glass bubble, flattening it out, and then cutting the biggest possible square from the resulting pancake, which was rarely more than a few inches on a side. A dozen or more such panes could be combined into a window using muntin bars to hold them in place. These panes are called "lights" because for a long time that's about all they were good for: too small and ripply to offer views of any consequence, their main purpose was illumination.

In early American houses, window lights were few and far between. Most glass came from England, and during the Colonial period windowpanes were heavily taxed. Before improvements in the design of fireplaces, the light that windows offered also had to be weighed against the draughts of cold air they admitted. Not that anyone at the time would have wanted even a Thermopaned picture window, assuming such a thing had been within the grasp of technology: the taste for looking at landscape, which was an invention of the romantics, still lay in the future. And in America, where the outdoors was still regarded as a howling wilderness, the haunt of Satan and Indians and abominable weather, the desire to gaze out of a window, except for the purpose of spying a threat, was slight, or nil. Refuge in those days counted for more than prospect.

Indeed, the early Colonial window, with its high proportion of wood to glass and its parsimonious admission of light, was probably a fair reflection of the prevailing attitude toward the world outside. Medieval Christianity, as well as Puritanism, drew a sharp line between the spiritual sanctuary provided by interiors and the profanity of the outdoor world. When the world beyond the window consists of so much peril (spiritual and otherwise), that window is apt to be small and difficult to open.

The development of clear, leaded glass in 1674, followed a century later by sheet glass made with iron rollers, coincided with—and no doubt helped to promote—important changes in people's attitude toward the world beyond the window. Beginning with the Enlightenment, people were less inclined to regard the world outside as perilous or profane; indeed, nature itself now became the site of spiritual sanctuary, the place one went to find oneself, as Rousseau would do on his solitary walks. Nature became the remedy for a great many ills, both physical and spiritual, and the walls that divided us from its salubrious effects came to be seen as unwelcome barriers. As Richard Sennett suggests in a fascinating study of perception and social life called *The Conscience of the Eye*, transparency—of self to nature, of self to other—became a high Enlightenment ideal. Writes Sennett, "The Enlightenment conceived a person's inner life opened up to the environment as though one had flung a window open to fresh air."

Sentiments of this kind, abetted by improvements in glassmaking, led to a dramatic increase in the size of windowpanes and sash over the course of the eighteenth century. The floor-to-ceiling casements known as French windows, which first appeared at Versailles in the 1680s, became popular on both sides of the Atlantic during this period (Jefferson installed several of them at Monticello), as did the gigantic double-hung windows that the Dutch invented around the same time to light the interiors of their long, narrow homes. Muntin bars were still commonly used in windows, but for a new purpose: They helped distribute the weight of the panes, thereby making it possible to build much larger windows. Beyond providing air and light, windows now admitted the landscape to the interior of a house.

A line of historical descent can be drawn from the Enlightenment window to the modernist glass wall, and Sennett draws a convincing one, passing through the great Victorian greenhouses—the first vast spaces to be enclosed in glass, creating the novel sensation of being at once indoors and outdoors—on its way to the Bauhaus's curtain walls and the glass houses built by Mies van der Rohe and Philip Johnson. But it seems to me this line of historical development spent at least part of the nineteenth century in America, passing close by Concord, where Emerson was imagining himself a "transparent eyeball" in Nature, and Walden Pond, where Henry Thoreau was giving voice to the dream of a transparent habitation.

The fenestration of Thoreau's own cabin was nothing special: the sole double-hung window that punctuated the long wall where he kept his writing table probably did little to relieve the interior gloom of the house at Walden. But Thoreau's imaginary architecture was way out ahead of what he actually managed to build, and it proved by far the more influential. You'll recall how he waited until the latest possible moment that first fall to plaster his cabin walls, so much did he enjoy the transit of breezes through his building's frame, "so slightly clad." Sworn enemy of walls and bounds and frames of any kind, he declared that his favorite "room" at Walden was the pine wood outside his door, swept clean by that "priceless domestic," the wind. In a memorable passage, he described cleaning day at Walden, when he moved his writing table and all his household effects outside on the grass, turning his house inside out. "It was worth the while to see the sun shine on these things," he wrote, "and hear the free wind blow on them; so much more interesting most familiar objects look out of doors than in the house."

Thoreau's dream of a house utterly transparent to nature, one in which the usual distinctions between indoors and out have been erased, is a beguiling one, and no doubt lies somewhere in back of my wish for a building that could be turned into a porch any time summer afforded me a benign enough afternoon. It probably lies behind Philip Johnson's glass house too, whose transparency does not so much destroy all sense of enclosure as extend it to the tree line outside, which becomes the house's true walls.

In the twentieth century, the ideal of transparency became closely bound up with the whole utopian project of modernism, and it embraced a great deal more than nature. Modernist architecture sought, too, a transparency of construction (hence no trim) and function (no ornament) and space (no interior walls). Since transparency implied truthfulness and freedom, and opacity suggested deception, it was perhaps inevitable that glass would emerge as the supreme modernist material—though "material" is perhaps too stingy and earthbound a word for everything that glass represented in the modernist imagination. Far from being a mere building material, plate glass offered nothing less than the means for building a new man and a new society, one in which transparency would break down once and for all the barriers that divide us one from another, as well as from nature. Seemingly the most modern and least haunted of materials, glass promised to deliver humanity from the burden of its past and equip it for a shining future.

In 1914 a German engineer and science fiction writer named Paul Scheerbart extolled the millennial promise of glass in a rhapsodic manifesto:

We mostly inhabit closed spaces. These form the milieu from which our culture develops. . . . If we wish to raise our culture to a higher plane, so must we willy-nilly change our architecture. And that will be possible only when we remove the sense of enclosure from the spaces where we live. And this we will only achieve by introducing Glass Architecture.

Scheerbart went on to predict that the word *Fenster* was about to vanish from the dictionary, as windows gave way to glass walls.

The artists and architects of the Bauhaus took this man for a prophet. Even the Marxist critic Walter Benjamin, a fervent admirer, championed the glass cause, declaring that "to live in a glass house is a revolutionary virtue par excellence. It is also an intoxication, a moral exhibitionism, that we badly need." The absolute exposure guaranteed by glass would purge society of its ills like a cleansing blast of light and fresh air. Some went so far as to claim that glass architecture heralded the end of war, on the theory that people in glass houses would know better than to throw stones (a transparent-enough *idea*, anyway). For a time, glass was invested with the sort of mystical significance and magical possibility that for most of history has swirled around gold.

It was structural steel that made glass architecture something more than the dream of socialists and science fiction writers. Since the birth of architecture, the size of windows—and especially their horizontal extent—has been constrained by the load-bearing function of the wall; many of the great innovations in architecture—such as the Gothic arch and the flying buttress—have had as their aim the freeing of walls so that they might hold bigger windows. If the history of architecture truly was, as Le Corbusier wrote, "the struggle for the window," then with the invention of structural steel, that struggle was won. No longer needed to support the weight of the floors, walls could now hold vast horizontal expanses of undivided plate glass. (Needless to say, the muntin bar—being no longer functional, and hopelessly old-fashioned—didn't stand a

chance with the modernists.) With a further assist from the eleva-
tor (glass walls being easier to live with high up in the sky) and the
air conditioner, glass architecture now leapt off the drafting table.

But in practice glass architecture was full of unexpected and not
altogether pleasant ironies, some of which undoubtedly prepared
the way for the return of the muntin and the traditional window. As
anyone who's spent any time behind the curtain wall of an office
building could tell you, plate glass was discomfiting in ways the
theories hadn't anticipated. One felt exposed and vulnerable behind a wall of glass. Some claimed this was a vestigial, bourgeois
sentiment that people would eventually outgrow, as "moral exhibitionism" caught on. But there was another problem. Instead of
connecting people to what lies beyond it, plate glass seemed to do
the very opposite, to evoke a sense of alienation. The glass wall had
an unexpected way of distancing you from the world on the other
side, from "the view."

The exigencies of glass construction were partly to blame: glass
walls, and even the "picture windows" that soon emerged as the
glass architecture of the common man, had to be extra-thick for
strength and double- or triple-glazed for insulation. Since such "windows" were obviously too large and heavy to be opened, the practical
effect of glass architecture, as Sennett points out, was to achieve a
transparency that was strictly *visual*. Not that this troubled the modernists, many of whom belonged to a long tradition in the West of fa-
voring the eye over the other senses. The eye, Le Corbusier had
declared, was "the master of ceremonies" in architecture; sometimes
in his sketches he would draw an eyeball as a stand-in for the occu-
pant of a house. Yet without the additional information provided by
the senses of smell and touch and hearing, the world as perceived
through a plate of glass can seem profoundly, and disconcertingly,
inaccessible. More so, even, than the world beyond a wall of wood or
stone, perhaps because the transparency promised by glass arouses
sensory expectations that the material can't fulfill.

At street level too, plate glass proved unexpectedly alienating, inside as well as out. During the day, the glass building was scarcely transparent at all, and its reflectivity often made it an aloof and ghostly presence on the street. Faceless, cold, it seemed constitutionally incapable of making any connection with its surroundings, except to mirror them, mutely.

The wall of glass itself created a powerful social barrier that its champions had failed to foresee; to the extent that glass facilitated a "moral exhibitionism," this was not a pretty or uplifting sight to behold. There are avenues in midtown Manhattan—Park in the Fifties, say, or Madison in the Sixties and Seventies—lined with posh shops and banks and galleries where the wall of plate glass at street level serves to isolate those well heeled enough to be buzzed in as effectively as a castle moat. There is one particular block in the Fifties on Sixth Avenue, the Manhattan thoroughfare that gave itself most wholeheartedly to modernism, where a homeless woman can gaze up and watch a famous magazine publisher making deals behind the glass wall of his second-story corner office: there's the phone pressed to the ear, the hand gestures, the suit jacket draped over the arm of the sofa. The only reason I know about this homeless woman is that I was once inside this particular office, and briefly caught her eye, across the gulf of glass. It was a connection, I suppose, but not the kind that the modernists had prophesied.

If plate glass in the city tended to underscore the distances between people, in the suburbs and the countryside its effects were less brutal but no more socially constructive. In the suburbs the picture window, in search of a suitably picturesque view, tended to turn the attention of the houses away from the street, where the front porch had fixed it, and back toward the landscape. Magazines such as *House Beautiful* published articles on how to avoid the "fishbowl effect" of picture windows by planting hedges out front or restricting them to the backyard; either way, the large expanses of undivided glass tended to avert one's gaze from the neighbors and the street, furthering privacy at the expense of community.

Most modernist houses were designed for (if not always built in) the sort of unpeopled rural landscapes where transparency promised to be somewhat more congenial to the homeowner. If the mass-market picture window took one's eyes off the street, the genuine modernist article—the glass walls and *fenêtres en longueur*—was inconceivable unless you owned the whole street or at least enough land to obliterate its presence. (Though even then, the sense of exposure is apparently hard to take: Philip Johnson doesn't actually *sleep* in his glass house, but in a cozy old Colonial down the road.) The modernist house with its glass walls is as impractical on a small plot of land as a picturesque garden with its ha-ha: Both require large and isolated holdings for the proper functioning of their transparencies.

So much for the glass utopia.

≡

Like most people, I have never actually lived in a glass house, but when I was a boy my parents built a summer home at the shore whose design, I realize now, was beholden to the modernist dream of transparency. My father designed it himself with the help of a contractor, which suggests just how general some of these ideas had become by 1965. The house was a modified A-frame built on an open plan, with kitchen, living room, and dining room all flowing together, and its front wall, which looked out at the Atlantic Ocean, was almost entirely glazed: There were sliding glass doors on one side, a big horizontal picture window on the other, and above, undivided plates of glass rising all the way up into the peak. A half-dozen other houses were similarly deployed along a strip of sand dune, and together they resembled a flock of weathered gray birds perched on a wire, all staring intently ahead. Indeed, our house had only a couple of windows

on its side walls, and these were cheap little double-hungs, strictly for ventilation. It was the big view that my parents had bought,
and it was the big view and nothing else that their house was
going to look at.

What I remember about our glass wall and its big view (besides
the fact that the living room was always too hot and you never entered it except fully dressed, even though the only creature apt to
look in was a gull) was that the ocean view was best appreciated
from the couch, as if you were watching a movie—which the proportions, or "aspect ratio," of the picture window closely approxi-
mated. It must be a convention of our visual culture that an image
of roughly these proportions says, "Look no further: Here's the
whole picture," because I can't remember ever feeling the urge to
get up from the couch for a closer look. A smaller or squarer window, on the other hand, seems to invite us to step up to it and
peak out, glimpse what lies beyond the frame on either side. Every
opening in a wall proposes a certain amount of mystery, and this
is directly proportional to its size, with "keyhole" at one end of the
scale. But a big window, and especially a big horizontal window,
offers no more or different information when your nose is pressed
against it than it does from a distance, so why get up? Like the
single-point perspective of a Renaissance painting, the picture
window posits an unmoving eye situated at a specific point in
space, and this might as well be coordinated with the location of
a particularly comfortable sofa.

My parents' view also acquainted me with the peculiar distancing effect of plate glass. Ours was double-glazed, and unless the
big slider had been left ajar, the seal of the wall was complete. You
saw the waves break white out beyond the dunes, but heard nothing; watched the sea grass bend and flash under the breeze, but
felt nothing. There was a deadness to it, a quality of having already
happened. The view seemed far away, static, and inaccessible, except of course to the eye.

Our picture window's horizontal format probably contributed to this impression. As painters understand, the horizontal dimension is the eye's natural field of play, the axis along which it ordinarily takes in the world. Compared to a vertical format, which is more likely to engage the whole body, inviting the viewer into the picture as if through a door, the horizontal somehow seems cooler, disembodied, more cerebral. This might be because people seem instinctively to project themselves into the spaces they see, and we don't imagine our upright bodies passing through a horizontal opening, just our eyes, and possibly our minds.

Only much later did I realize that my parents' picture window contained its own implicit philosophy of nature, one perhaps not quite as benign as its sheer appreciativeness might suggest. True, compared to the attitude of fear or antagonism toward the outdoors implied by the small pre-Enlightenment window, the picture window tells a considerably friendlier story about nature. Yet to put nature up on a kind of pedestal, as the picture window does, is to hold it at arm's length, regard it as an aesthetic object—a "picture." Our sole involvement with it is the gaze, which is fixed, cool, timeless, and possessive. (For this is "our" view, and we resent anybody who tampers with it.) The picture window turns the stuff of nature into a *landscape*, the very idea of which implies separation and observation and passivity—nature as spectator sport, which suited my father the indoorsman just fine.

Of course, the rural picture window doesn't make a picture out of any old stretch of nature. Nobody ever placed one directly in front of a group of trees or the face of a boulder, and my parents never thought to put theirs on the wall that faced a pretty grove of gnarled beetlebung trees. No, a picture window must give the horizon its due, and the content of the view will always be something "special," by which we usually mean "picturesque." The space invariably will be deep (divided into near, middle, and far); the land pristine and changeless (except for the effects of weather and seasons), and there will be few if any signs of human work.

Implied in the very idea of a picture window is an assumption that there is a "special" nature that is entitled to our gaze and care, and an ordinary nature that is not. In this the picture window is in tune ideologically with tourism and environmentalism, both of which lavish their attention on those landscapes that most nearly resemble wilderness—places unpeopled, timeless, and pristine; nature *out there*—at the expense of all those ordinary places where most of us live and work, and which may be just as deserving of our attention and care. There might be some kind of window that discloses the beauty of such places, but it is not a picture window.

Though a picture window obviously has a frame (you can't have a window or even a glass wall without one), it pretends otherwise. A frame always implies a point of view, the presence of some ordering principle or sensibility. Yet by eliminating muntins (which call attention to the sash) and stretching out horizontally to the peripheries of our field of vision, the picture window suggests that its view of nature is perfectly objective and unmediated: *This is it, how it really is out there.* And the full-scale glass wall goes even further, dropping the "out there" from the claim, since now any distance between ourselves and nature has supposedly been eliminated. If the picture window resembles a pair of eyeglasses so large the wearer loses sight of the frame, the glass house is a contact lens. The conceit of its more radical transparency is that the frame can be eliminated, leaving us with a perfect apprehension of nature, a clear seeing with nothing interposed save this inconsequential pane of glass—whose own reality everything has been done to suppress.

But perhaps the tallest tale told by plate glass is of man's power and nature's benignity. The promise of modernity was that we could master nature with our technology and science, and what better way to express that mastery—flaunt it, even—than building houses made of glass? Humankind has outgrown the need for refuge, the glass house says; now prospect alone can rule architecture. I was reminded of the ridiculousness of this particular conceit every time the weather bureau issued a hurricane warning for our stretch of Atlantic seaboard. My father and I would scamper up ladders to crisscross the great glass wall with webs of masking tape. The tape was supposed to help the glass withstand the gales, and these flimsy paper muntins did somehow make us feel marginally safer as the wind blew. After a few years of hurricane alerts, the glass wall had been scarred by the fossil traces of tape glue, an abiding rebuke to its boast of transparency.

≡

While waiting for Jim Evangelisti to finish and truck over the windows, Joe and I spent a couple of Saturdays building the four small peak windows. Charlie hadn't drawn these units in any detail, so fabricating and designing them proceeded hand in hand. We decided on a narrow stock for our windows—one-by-one pine for the sash; three-quarter-inch for the casing—since our rough openings were only a foot square and I wanted as big a pane of glass as possible. Following Jim's example, we drew a full-scale diagram of the windows on a sheet of oak tag; this became a template for the dozens of precisely dimensioned pieces of pine we needed to cut.

I manned the table saw, cutting strips of pine to length and mitering their ends, while Joe handled the more sensitive routing work, making the grooves that would hold our glass and form our joints. Since two of the windows were to be operable (one at either end of the building, for ventilation), the frame of their sash needed a sturdy joint that could be counted on to hold its right angles indefinitely; only a sash that remained perfectly true would open reliably and keep out the rain. After we fit the pieces together and checked the frames for square, we glued the corners, resquared and clamped the assembly, and then tacked the joints with brads for good measure.

After the frames had dried, I attached them to their casing with hinges and then attempted to glaze the sash, a process that did indeed require a certain knack, as Jim had mentioned. The window-pane is held in place with a beveled bead of glazing putty, which is applied to the corner where it meets the wood frame with a putty knife that must be wielded at a precise forty-five-degree angle. Move the knife too slowly and the putty blobs up on you; move it too fast and it tears. Turning corners neatly is the real test, though, requiring skill and a bit of nerve. By the time I'd glazed my fourth window, I could manage a respectable straightaway, but my corners remained somewhat bulbous.

Luckily for me these windows would be twelve feet off the ground, so no one would ever be in a position to observe the gentleness of my learning curve. I took heart in what I'd read about the Arts and Crafts movement's liberal line on mistakes: "There is hope in honest error," one designer had declared, "none in the icy perfections of the mere stylist." Small mistakes in the finished product revealed the hand of the worker; perfection was opaque. Certainly the mark of my own unhandy hands was visible in these windows, which were hopeful in the extreme. Joe held up one of the finished sashes to his face and peered out at me through its frame. "It's a window." This was about all you could say for it, apart from the fact it was the absolutely squarest thing Joe and I had so far managed to build.

Jim delivered his own rather more accomplished windows on Christmas Eve, and Joe and I had them all installed by the end of an unseasonably warm New Year's Day, a swift and hugely satisfying process that revolutionized the building both inside and out. Since Jim had already put on the hinges and painted the sash (a deep blackish green), installation was basically a matter of squaring and plumbing each casing in its rough opening in the wall, then securing it to the frame and hanging the sash.

And on an ordinary building this would have been a snap. But since ninety degrees was not this particular building's predominant angle (no blaming Charlie for that one), we struggled for a while trying to determine exactly what plane each window should occupy in its wall; our rough openings were *rough*. After some adjustments and difference-splitting, we slipped the window casings into their openings. Shimming them with scraps of leftover shingle, we'd nudge the jambs a fraction of an inch this way or that and then, after consulting the level and the square, lock the right angle into place with a long galvanized wood screw. It was right here that the ever-widening gyre of oblique and obtuse angles that had bedeviled the construction from the start was finally halted; had it not been, my windows would never have closed properly. Now we lifted each sash into its casing, interlocked the knuckles on each half of hinge, and then inserted the brass pin that held the two halves together. The windows were in.

From the outside, the building was suddenly much more interesting to look at—because now the building looked back. It had a face. Roused by glass from its long material slumber, the structure now seemed something more than the sum of its wooden parts, as though, Oz-like, it had been inspirited. Especially after we'd installed the two windows in the peak, from which they peered out with a supervisory air, the building looked, if not alive, then at least like a pretty good metaphor for consciousness, with its big awning windows reflecting back the landscape in what seemed almost a form of acknowledgment. Like water in the landscape, which is likewise reflective and transparent by turns, glass has a way of inflecting whatever holds it, quickening what was formerly inert, suggesting other layers and dimensions, depths to plumb. And though I'm sure a big pane of plate glass would have animated the building too, I doubt it would have made it look nearly as, well, *smart* as my building now seemed. (Joe said the little windows up in the peak had given the building its brains.) Undivided plates of glass often wear a glazed expression, look blind. Muntins wink.

Inside too, the windows had invested the building with a kind of intelligence, a point of view. What had been a single uninflected horizontal view out over the desk was now divided into six discrete square frames. The surprise was just how much more you could see this way, now that there were six focal points instead of one, and twenty-four edges composing the scene instead of four. Here, top center, was a picture of the white oak, holding a great bowl of space in its bare upturned arms. Below it was a frame of vegetable garden blasted by winter; another of the iced pond, a glistening white tablet pressed into the freezer-burned earth; and, in the third, a trio of slender tree trunks leaning into the frame from off-stage, almost close enough to touch. I don't think I'd ever noticed these particular trees before; they were exactly the sort of ordinary, near-distance imagery we automatically edit out of a panoramic view. For someone not blessed with great powers of visual observation, the grid of muntin bars was a lesson in looking, a little like the graph paper art students sometimes use to break a scene down into manageable components.

I noticed that any movement on my part would radically revise the content of the six frames; the fixed point perspective of the undivided rough opening (much like a conventional picture window's) had given way to a shifting mosaic of views. Standing up on the landing, the view was strictly middle distance, looking down to the massive trunk of the white ash rising out of a chaotic, unmade bed of boulders. Only when you stepped down into the main room did the full picturesque prospect, with its deep and orderly space, pop into view. I thought of Charlie's metaphor of the prescription glasses, because the sensation recalled how putting on a fresh pair can snap the world so vividly into focus. I realized that Charlie had put the central window just where he had—down low over the desk—in order to seduce me into taking my seat, since there is where the prospect was most pleasing.

I knew this because I'd brought a chair out to the building to get some idea what working in front of this window would be like. It was the same chair I'd stood on back when I was deciding on the site, and now I slid it up to a chalked line representing the edge of my as-yet-unbuilt desk and sat down. This turned out to be the only spot in the room from which I could readily pop open and peer out of the little recessed window directly to my right—yet another way Charlie had deployed his windows to lure me to my desk. We seem to gravitate naturally toward windows (Christopher Alexander says this is because we're "phototropic"), and Charlie was using this fact to organize my experience of the room.

This particular window reminded me of the little triangular smoking windows cars used to have up front, or the side window in a prop plane's cockpit, the one the pilot slides open to receive the manifest from the ground crew. My own cockpit window overlooked the big rock, making for a decidedly unpicturesque view, all jammed up with the muscled back of a boulder not three feet away. This particular frame was like a blown-up photograph, a detail dwelling on the intricate map of lichens and moss that covered the granite skin. The view was utterly bereft of prospect; it told of rootedness and refuge instead, not at all what you expect from a window.

And yet it was perfectly in keeping with the building's *parti*, the two thick walls giving refuge side to side while the thin ones, which seemed even thinner now that they'd been glazed and delicately subdivided with muntins, opened up to prospect fore and aft. Across the room the other thick wall was now pierced by a French casement that opened on no "view" at all but a latticework of cedar. In a year's time this trellis would be draped in leaves and the casement would open directly on a second and entirely different image of refuge: the gardener's hedgey green wall, no farther away than your nose.

Behind me the big awning looked up the hill toward the meadow, which seemed to tumble down toward it, and, high above, the two peak windows on either gable each admitted a paragraph of sky—just enough light to flatter Charlie's boat-hull ceiling, throwing its rhythms of wood into relief and coloring its fir straps blood orange. Though all the new windows were badly smudged, and the early winter sun was feeble, the little room was awash in a light that already seemed its own.

Naturally I had to test out the operation of my windows too. Each of them had its own custom operating system (tracking down workable hardware for these had been almost as difficult as finding the drip edge detail). What came as news to me was the way a particular arrangement of hinges and handles on a sash could call forth a particular physical gesture in the act of opening it, engaging the body in a very specific way. This building now summoned a whole vocabulary of these gestures, and each expressed a slightly different attitude toward the world outdoors. It was something an actor would have grasped immediately, how, say, hoisting one of the big awning sashes and hooking it to its chain (they hung from a chrome chain suspended from the ridge beam) felt like lifting a garage door overhead and heading out into the bright workaday morning, or maybe it was more like propping up the wooden flaps on your root beer stand—another hopeful A.M. gesture that said OPEN FOR BUSINESS. Whereas pushing open the rock window, which was hinged on the side and swung out like some kind of utility door, had something distinctly hatchlike and vehicular about it: You almost wanted to reach out and give somebody the old thumbs-up before shoving off. As for the French casement on the south wall, this window opened in an altogether different and more genteel world—a bedroom, say, or kitchen—and the action of its sash called for a refined, even feminine gesture, two hands drawing the day in like a breath. This window you could open in your pj's, where the side window called for a uniform, maybe, or jumpsuit.

However attired, I could see that opening up and closing this building was definitely not going to be a swift or simple operation. For one thing, the procedure had to be executed in the correct sequence, always opening the French casement *after* raising the awning, lest the swinging sashes collide. It looked like summer mornings were going to enlist me in a skippery ritual of rigging and tacking the various parts of my building, and then at day's end performing the reverse operation, carefully stowing everything and battening down the hatches, my own landlocked rendition of the seafarer's rigmarole. One thing this building's attitude toward the world outside its windows would *not* be was passive.

≡

So what story did my windows have to tell, about nature and our relationship to it? The answer to this question eluded me at first, perhaps because the pictures of nature my windows offered were so various that they seemed to defy generalization. One frame might attend to the picturesque while another threw that whole idea into question, making a nice case for nature's unspectaculars: the anonymous trees and weeds and ho-hum topographies of the middle distance. And still others had little use for pictures at all, preferring instead to snag a northerly breeze or wedge of overhead light. But maybe that *was* the point, or if not the point (for I doubt Charlie intended it) then at least the effect: to suggest that nature might be more various than any one of our conceptions of it. That any single view—whether it be wilderness or garden, sublime or picturesque, refuge or prospect—is only that, a version of nature and not the whole of it.

In place of the single, steady gaze, the room proposes a multitude of glimpses, and these are so different one from the next that sometimes it's hard to believe a single tiny room that *wasn't* a vehicle could supply them all. The picture of nature on offer here seems partial, mobile, and cumulative, built up not only from glances and gazes but also from the various bodily sensations that opening a particular window can provide, beginning with the feel of a handle's grip and ending with a sample of the afternoon air. And every one of them is distinct—not only the view but the grip and even the air, whose scent and weight seem to shift with the cardinal points. And come summer, when I move into full porch mode, throwing the house as open as a gazebo or belvedere to the breeze and rush of space, the picture of nature on offer here will be more layered and complicated still. "Picture" won't even be the word for it.

But then what about the word "transparency"? Surely that is part of the story these custom windows have to tell, with their in-swinging sash that can open the better part of a wall to the outdoor air. This is not, however, the transparency of a modernist, fooling the eye with an illusion of framelessness, so much as the qualified and much more sensual transparency of the porch. A porch is always frankly framed, as my building will be, by its thick, heavy walls, the ever-present ceiling, and the wooden visor in front that, like the visor on a cap, is a constant reminder that something's been edited out, that here is one perspective. Rather than pretend to framelessness, to objectivity, opening all my windows will turn this whole building into a frame.

The romantics and the modernists were right to suspect the window frame of standing between ourselves and nature, between us and others, but I suspect they were probably wrong to think this distance could ever be closed. It won't be, not by glass walls, not by flinging windows wide open, not even by blowing up the houses. For even outdoors, even in the pine wood that Thoreau said was his favorite room at Walden, we are still in some irreducible sense outside nature. As *Walden* itself teaches us, we humans are never simply in nature, like the beasts and trees and boulders, but are always also *in relation* to nature: looking at it through the frames of our various preconceptions, our personal and collective histories, our self-consciousness, our words. There might be value in breaking frames and pushing toward transparency, as Thoreau and his fellow romantics (the Zen masters too) have urged us to do, but the goal is probably beyond our reach. What other creature, after all, even *has* a relationship to nature? The window, with its qualified transparency and its inevitable frame, is the sign of this fact of relation, of difference.

This was, for me, a slightly melancholy discovery, since it had been in quest of a certain transparency that I'd set out on this journey. By building this house off in the woods, and by making it with my own hands, I'd hoped to break out of a few of the frames that stood between me and experience, especially the panes of words that boxed in so much of my time and attention and seemed to distance me from the world of things and the senses. Though I suppose I had accomplished this, it seemed clear now that what I'd really done was trade some old frames for a few new ones. Which might be the best we can hope for, transparency being as elusive as truth. Not that the trying wasn't worth the effort; it was. Just look at what I had to show for it: this building and these new windows, for one thing, which have given me so much more than a view. And then there were the new and sometimes warring perspectives I'd acquired along the way—that of carpenter and architect, I mean, not to mention apprentice; there were all those new windows too. Maybe it wasn't as important to see things as they "really" are as it was to see them freshly, scrupulously, and from more than one point of view.

Charlie had been right all along about going custom. To do so might not be straightforward or cheap, yet clearly it is possible to improve on the standard windows, these ways of seeing we've inherited. Some windows *are* better than others, can cast the world in a fresher light, even make it new. As Charlie said, you can pick up a pair of glasses at Woolworth's, or you can spring for a prescription.

Yet there is still and always the frame, even if one has perfect vision and sleeps out under the stars. Transparency's for the birds, for them and all the rest of nature. As for us, well, we do windows.

CHAPTER 8

Finish Work:
A Punch List

Once we'd butted the last course of shingles tight
to the window casings and squeezed a bead of
caulk along the joint, the building was at last
sealed to the weather and Joe and I could start in
on finish work. To my ear, the term had a welcome, auspicious ring, signifying as it did that we
were moving indoors (it was January now, deep
winter) and toward completion. This showed just
how little I understood about the meaning of finish work, however, for nothing else in house building takes quite as long. I automatically assumed
the primary meaning of the term to be temporal
(*Hey, we must be nearly finished!*), but of course
finishing in carpentry also has a spatial meaning,
having to do with an exalted level of refinement in

the joining and dressing of interior wood. In fact, this turns out to be so time-consuming it's apt to make finishing in the other sense of the word seem like a receding, ungraspable mirage.

Progress slows. Or at least it appears to, since it is by now such a subtle thing, measured in increments of smoothness and crafts-manship and in to-do lists done rather than in changes at the scale of a landscape or elevation. No one big thing, finish work consists of a great variety of discrete tasks, many niggling, some inspiring, but none you would call heroic. And yet, day by day, each task checked off moves you another notch down the punch list, that much closer to move-in day, when the time of building ends and the time of habitation begins. Joe and I would spend the better part of a year finishing the writing house.

Framing by comparison is epic work—the raising from the ground of a whole new structure in a matter of days. There's poetry in finish work too, but it's a small, domestic sort of poetry, which I suppose is appropriate enough. Building the desk, trimming out the windows, sanding and rubbing oil into wood surfaces to raise their grain and protect them, is slow, painstaking work that seems to take place well out of earshot of the gods. High ritual might at-tend the raising of a ridge beam, but who ever felt the need to bless a baseboard molding, or say a little prayer over the punch list?

No, finish work takes place in the realm of the humanly visible and tactile, and it is chiefly this that accounts for its laboriousness. Its concern is with the intimate, inescapable surfaces of everyday life—the desk one faces each morning, with its achingly familiar wood-grain figures, the sill on which an elbow or coffee cup habit-ually rests—and any lapse of attention here will leave its mark, if not on the land, then certainly on the texture of a few thousand days. Where being off by an eighth or a sixteenth of an inch was good enough when we were nailing shingles or spacing two-by-fours, the acceptable margins of error and imperfection had by now dwindled to nothing. Now we dealt in thirty-seconds of an inch, and strove for "drive fits" in wood joints that take the tap of a mallet to secure; now even hairline gaps rankle, and at close quarters indoors the eye can distinguish eighty-eight degrees from ninety. Fortunately one's education in carpentry follows a course that makes the achievement of such exactitude at least theoretically plausible. Each stage in the building process demands a progressively higher level of refinement and skill, as the novice moves from framing to cladding to shingling and then finally to finish work, so that at this point in the construction I should have hammered enough nails and cut enough lengths of lumber to know how to do the job right. Theoretically.

Owing to the peculiarities of Charlie's design, the finish work called for in my building was not "normal," in Joe's estimation. In some ways it was more challenging than the usual—there were all the built-ins to be built (the desk, the daybed, the shelves), and an "articulated" structure such as this always makes it more difficult for the carpenter to cover his tracks with trim or wallboard, carpentry's blessed absolutions. But in other ways the finish work promised to be relatively simple—a little *too* simple, as far as Joe was concerned. Finish is where a carpenter usually gets to show off his craftsmanship, and Charlie hadn't left much scope for the exercise of Joe's virtuosity with the jigsaw or router.

The plans called for a bare minimum of trim, for example, and what there was of it was fairly straightforward—not an ogee, fillet, or coping in sight. Only a small section of the walls—the area immediately surrounding the daybed—would be closed in, with narrow boards of clear white pine. The windows were supposed to be trimmed out with one-inch strips of the same clear pine, just enough to bridge the quarter-inch gap between post and casing. There were no baseboard moldings, unless you count the Doug-fir kick plate facing the bottommost bookshelf. And the plywood-and-two-by-four fin walls that held the bookshelves were to be sanded and oiled but left untrimmed: the "ornament" here, such as it was, consisted of the way the vertical two-by-four at the front of each fin wall came three-quarters of an inch proud of the exposed edge of the plywood that faced its sides.

At least since the day that modernism turned Viennese architect Adolph Loos's silly declaration that "ornament is crime" into a battle cry, the whole issue of trim has been a heated one in architecture, and Joe's and my differences in outlook on this question were bound to come to a head sooner or later. On the one and only day Joe worked on the building by himself (I was out of town), he trimmed out a pair of the little peak windows with a fancy picture-frame molding, an expertly mitered piece of handiwork he was tremendously proud of. The day I got back he phoned to see what I thought of it. It was true that the drawings were somewhat vague on Charlie's intention here, but it seemed to me Joe's solution was too decorative for this building, and I very gingerly told him so. It took two weeks and all the diplomatic skill I could muster before we could even talk about actually replacing it, and even then the discussion came down to his inevitable half-surly, half-sulking shrug of resignation and challenge: "Mike, it's your building." But for some reason this time around Joe's big line, calculated to put me on the defensive and check Charlie's authority, struck my ears differently than it had before. Had I said anything about Charlie? No!—it was by *my* lights that Joe's trim looked wrong. So, to put an end to the discussion, I simply said, "Joe, you're right: It *is* my building."

And yet it wasn't, not yet. Because although I'd worked on the building for more than two years, and although move-in day was in sight, the building still didn't feel like it was mine, not in any meaningful sense. I might have dreamed up the program and paid all the bills, but this was Charlie's design we had been building, and, let's face it, even now I would be lost without Joe's help—it was doubtful I could finish alone. For very good reasons, Joe and Charlie both seemed to feel more proprietary about the building than I did—which is why the two of them were by this point incapable of exchanging an untesty word. But in all the time I'd spent mediating their warring claims, I hadn't really ever asserted my own.

There was some sort of key to the building that was still missing, I felt, something that was needed in order to make it truly mine, and I began to wonder if this key might not have to do with time. Finishing didn't mean the same thing to Joe and Charlie as it did to me: I wasn't going to be finished with this building the day the building inspector wrote out the certificate of occupancy and the two of them headed home for the last time, turning over this page in their lives; nor was the building going to be finished with me. I alone would be accompanying it into the future, and it would be accompanying me. A not un-obvious thought, perhaps, yet it helped me to appreciate that the last thing these last surfaces and their finishes were was "superficial"; they were precisely where the building and I would spend the next however-many years rubbing up against one another, and possibly even rubbing off. Made right, these walls, this floor, this desk, might someday come to fit me as well as an old pair of shoes, be just as expressive of my daily life; feel as much mine, I mean, as a second skin. Yet is it possible to *make* such a thing? I wasn't sure, but if it was, I decided, it would involve paying some closer attention—even now, before it was finished—to the life of the building in time.

✓ TIME AND PLACE

Time is not something architects talk about much, except in the negative. The common view seems to be that mortal time is what buildings exist to transcend; being immortal (at least compared to their builders), buildings give us a way to leave a lasting mark, to conduct a conversation across the generations, in Vincent Scully's memorable formulation. I doubt there are many builders or architects in history who would dispute Le Corbusier's dictum that the first aim of architecture is to defy time and decay—to make something in space that time's arrow cannot pierce.

Or even scuff, in the case of Le Corbusier and many of his contemporaries. The modernists were avid about making buildings that had as little to do with time as possible, time future as much as time past. That modernist buildings strove to sever their ties to history is well known. But if modernism was a dream of a house unhaunted by the past, its designers seemed equally concerned to inoculate their buildings against the future. They designed and built them in such a way as to leave as little scope as possible for the sort of changes that the passing of time has always wrought on a building—namely, the effects of nature outside, and of the owners within.

Defying the time of nature meant rejecting stone and wood, those symbols of the architectural past that have traditionally been prized for the graceful way they weather and show their age. Modernists preferred to clad their buildings in a seamless, white, and very often machined surface that was intended to look new forever. What this meant in practice, however, was an exterior that didn't so much weather as deteriorate, so that today the white building stained brown, by rust or air pollution, stands in most of the world's cities as a melancholy symbol of modernist folly. In architecture, time's objective correlative is grime.

Inside, too, modernists employed all sorts of novel, untested materials to which time has been unkind. But the important modernist attack on time indoors was less direct, and this had to do with human time, which in buildings takes the form of inhabitation. The modernists were the first architects in history to insist that they design the interiors of their houses down to the very last detail—not only the finish trims, which in the past had usually been left to the discretion of craftsmen, but the bookshelves and cabinets ("Farewell the chests of yesteryear," Le Corbusier declared), the furniture and window treatments, and even in some cases the light switches and teapots and ashtrays. "Built-ins" became the order of the day. Everything that was conceivably designable the architect now wanted to design, the better to realize his building's *Gestalt*, a German word for totality much bandied about in the Bauhaus. Had there been a way to somehow redesign the bodies of the inhabitants to fit in better with the *Gestalt* of their new house, no doubt these architects would have given it a try.

As it was, the architects fretted over what the owners would do to their works of art, which, most of them agreed, would never again be as perfect as the day before move-in day. It is this pristine moment that became—and remains—the all-important one for modern architecture: the day the finished but not-yet-inhabited building gets its picture taken, freezing it in time. After that, it's downhill. "Very few of the houses," Frank Lloyd Wright once complained, were "anything but painful to me after the clients moved in and, helplessly, dragged the horrors of the old order along after them."

What exactly does a totalitarian approach to the details of modern architecture have to do with time? Wright's "horrors of the old order" and Corbusier's "chests of yesteryear" give the game away. As inevitably as weathering, the process of inhabiting a space leaves the marks of time all over it, and so constitutes a declension from the architect's ideal. A house that welcomes our stuff—our furniture and pictures, our keepsakes and other "horrors"—is one that we have been invited in some measure to help create or finish; ultimately such a house will tell a story about us, individuals with a history.

Modernists often designed their interiors not so much for particular individuals as for Man; they regarded the addition of clients' stuff as a subtraction from a creation they thought of as wholly their own. This is one legacy of modernism that we have yet to overcome; our stuff, and in turn our selves, still very often have trouble gaining a comfortable foothold in a modern interior. Even now most of them seem designed to look their best uninhabited. Stewart Brand, the author of a recent book on preservation called *How Buildings Learn*, tells of asking one architect what he learned from revisiting his buildings. "Oh, you never go back," the architect said, surprised at the question. "It's too discouraging." For many contemporary architects, time is the enemy of their art.

In *The Timeless Way of Building*, Alexander writes that "those of us who are concerned with buildings tend to forget too easily that all the life and soul of a place . . . depend not simply on the physical environment, but on the pattern of events which we experience there"—everything from the transit of sunlight through a room to the kinds of things we habitually do in it. J. B. Jackson makes a similar point in his essay "A Sense of Place, a Sense of Time," where he argues that we pay way too much attention to the design of places, when it is what we routinely do in them that gives them their character. "It is our sense of time, our sense of ritual" and everyday occurrence, he writes, "which in the long run creates our sense of place."

Certainly when I think about spaces that I remember as having a strong sense of place, it isn't the "architecture" that I picture, the geometrical arrangements of wood and stone and glass, but such things as watching the world go by from the front porch of the general store in town, or the scuffle of ten thousand shoes making their way to work beneath Grand Central Station's soaring vault, or the guttering light of jack-o'-lanterns illuminating the faces of square dancers in a New England hayloft. The "design" of these places and the recurring events that give them their qualities—the spaces and the times—have grown together in such a way that it is impossible to bring one to mind without the other.

Jackson is doubtful that architects can *design* memorable places like these, at least on purpose; for him habitation will trump design every time, and that is how it should be. Certainly it is true that some of the best places are not made so much as remade, as people find new and unforeseen ways to inhabit them over time. Alexander, an architect himself, has more faith that an architect can design the "great good place," but not entirely by himself and probably not all at once. This is because no single individual can possibly know enough to make from scratch something as complex and layered and *thick* as a great place; for the necessary help, he will need to invoke the past, and also the future.

The first move is obvious enough: The architect borrows from the past by adapting successful patterns, the ones that have been proven to support the kind of life the place hopes to house—porches and watching the world go by, for example. But what about the time to come? There is of course the time of weathering: age seems to endear a building to people, to strengthen its sense of place, and the choice of materials can give an architect a way to either flout or abet this process. But it seems to me there is another, more profound way an architect can open a building to the impress of its future. Forswearing a totalitarian approach to its details, the architect can instead leave just enough play in his design for others to "finish it"—first the craftsmen, with their particular knowledge and sense of the place, and then the inhabitants, with their stuff and with the incremental changes that, over time, the distinctive grooves of their lives will wear into its surfaces and spaces. It may be that making a great place, as opposed to a mere building or work of architectural art, requires a collaboration not so much in space as over time.

✓ THE UNFINISHED HOUSE

For a long time after the renovation of our house was finished and Judith and I had moved back in, whenever Charlie came to visit he had a disconcerting habit of staring at the walls, absently. "What are you looking at?" I would ask, worried he had spotted some grave flaw in construction. "Oh, nothing . . . nothing," he'd blandly insist, and then rejoin the conversation for a while, until after a decent interval his gaze would once again float off, catching on the bookshelves, or the painting we'd hung in the breakfast room.

We realized eventually that it was our stuff he was staring at, and we began to kid him about it. Only with the greatest reluctance did he finally admit that the way we'd arranged our books and things on the living room shelves was, well, not quite how he'd imagined it. It seems we hadn't adjusted quite enough of the adjustable shelves, so that the living room wall didn't have the proper mix of big and little spaces; he could imagine a much more satisfactory rhythm of upright, leaning, and laying-down volumes, punctuated with the occasional lamp or picture frame. By giving us a whole wall with adjustable shelves, Charlie had given us the freedom to complete the design of the living room; now that we had, it was all he could do not to get up and finish the job himself. I told him I'd always thought the nice thing about freedom was that nobody could tell you what to do with it.

For the contemporary architect, trained as he is to think of himself as a species of modern artist, surrendering control of his creation is never easy, no matter what he professes to believe about the importance of collaboration. Even Christopher Alexander takes an authoritarian turn in the end, laying down inflexible rules for the minimum depth of a porch (six feet) or the maximum width of a piece of finish trim (one-half inch). There isn't an architect alive who doesn't approvingly quote Mies van der Rohe's line that "God is in the details" (never mind that most other people credit the line to Flaubert). What strikes me as odd about this aphorism as applied to architecture is not so much the apotheosis of the detail as its implied identification of the architect with God. Even Charlie, who resists the monomaniacal tendencies of his profession, fought Judith for more Charlie-designed built-ins (she prefers old furniture), left almost no wall space for paintings (Judith is a painter), and proposed that he design not only the closet doors and medicine cabinets and towel racks (all of which we agreed to) but also the toilet-paper holders (which is where we finally drew the line). Much as he might theoretically want to, the modern architect is loath to leave anything to chance or time, much less to the dubious taste of carpenters and clients.

A superficial glance at the blueprints for my writing house might lead one to conclude that it represents a stark example of totalitarian architecture. Not counting my chair, everything in it has been designed: the bookshelves, the daybed, the desk—all are built in. On the blueprints Charlie even sketched in the books on the shelves, as if to suggest the correct ratio of upright to sideways volumes (with a few casual leaners—at precisely sixty degrees—thrown in for good measure). But even though the plans are highly detailed, that conclusion would be incorrect. In ways I was just beginning to appreciate, he had left plenty of space in the design for the passing of time and the impress of craftsmanship and habitation to finish it. Joe had grasped this right away—that was what his window trim was all about.

Charlie's finicky drawings of them notwithstanding, my building's two thick walls were where its design was perhaps most open, if not to our craftsmanship, then to my inhabitation of the place. By sketching an arrangement of my books on his blueprints, Charlie wasn't so much trying to impose a shelving policy on me as he was tacitly acknowledging the crucial part my stuff would play in establishing the look and tone of this room.

That my books were an integral part of the interior design I understood as soon as Joe and I built the shelves. Though technically "finished," they didn't look at all that way; the long walls stacked with empty plywood cubicles seemed skeletal and characterless, blank. And the walls were going to remain blank until I'd filled them with my books and things; only then would the thick walls actually feel thick, would the building answer to Charlie's basic conception of it as "a pair of bookshelves with a roof over it."

And even then the building would continue to evolve in important ways, because most of the materials and finishes Charlie had specified were the kind that time conspicuously alters. Outside, the cedar shingles would gently silver as they weathered; more slowly, the skeleton of oiled fir inside promised to redden and warm, and the white pine walls and trim would eventually turn the color of parchment. Except for its windowpanes and hardware, the building was made entirely of wood, the material most tightly bound to time. Its grain records its past, ring by annual ring, and though the tree stops growing when it's cut, it doesn't stop developing and changing. "Acquiring character" is what we say it's doing, as a wood surface absorbs our oils and accumulates layers of grime, as it is dignified by use and time. I'd told Charlie in my first letter I wanted a building that was less like a house than a piece of furniture; he'd designed a place that promised to age like one.

✓ THE WRITING DESK

In the case of my writing desk, however, Charlie seemed to have pushed this whole notion of "acquiring character" a bit too far. He had specified we build the desk out of a thick slab of clear white pine. I hadn't paid much attention to the choice until I happened to mention it to Jim Evangelisti one afternoon in his shop and uncorked a gusher of antiarchitect invective along with a lecture on a few things about wood he felt I needed to know.

I'd returned to Jim's shop because he'd agreed to let me run my floorboards through his planer and joiner—no small favor, since the boards in question were more than two hundred years old and studded with iron nails hidden beneath a crust of grime. The boards had already done a stint as a barn floor somewhere—probably in a hayloft, Jim guessed, from the fact that the wood showed so little evidence of hoof traffic. These were stupendous pieces of pine; many of them were knotless and close to two feet wide, meaning they'd been cut from the kind of old-growth trees that survive in New England today chiefly as legends. My parents had found a stack of these boards in their barn and offered them to Judith and me when we were renovating the house; there'd been just enough left over to floor the writing house. The remaining boards were badly caked with dirt and coats of milk paint, however. I'd test-sanded a couple of them, but this had left the wood looking a bit too self-consciously rustic for a building that made no bones about being new. So I tried taking the boards down an eighth of an inch with a plane, where I found clean wood of a clarity and warmth I'd never seen before. It looked like pale honey, or tea.

As Jim and I ran the boards through his planer, raising a nasty plume of shavings that smelled as old as the world—a wild perfume of attic, must, fungus, and lilac—we sneezed and talked about woods. Jim said that the boards appeared to be mixed to him—some were white pine, but others looked more like yellow pine, a harder though less desirable Southern species. Knotty and prone to twisting, yellow pine is difficult to work and notoriously hard on tools. Jim mentioned in passing that he still occasionally heard an old-timer call the wood by its old nickname: "nigger pine." The label might not have struck a nineteenth-century ear quite as violently as it does ours, but it's a safe bet no flattery of the wood was intended.

Jim made it clear he thought building a desk out of white pine was nuts; "Only an architect . . ." etc., etc. The wood was just too soft, he said; in no time it would be nicked and pitted and horribly scratched. I'd actually once raised the issue of wear with Charlie, after Joe had mentioned something about it, but Charlie had been unconcerned; indeed, that was precisely the idea, he'd told me, to have a surface that would very rapidly acquire a history.

"Think of those great old marked-up wooden desks we had in elementary school," Charlie'd said, growing animated as he spoke. "Remember how you'd scratch your initials in them with a Bic pen, try to decipher what last year's kid had written. Every one of those desks told a story." It was a romantic notion, and I'd fallen for it. Jim didn't, however, and not only because he was a woodworker for whom the prospect of a perfectly good piece of furniture being gouged at by Bic-wielding schoolchildren held no romance whatsoever. A white pine desk was so soft, he said, that it would take the impression of a ballpoint through several sheets of paper, which was more history than I probably wanted. I'd be unable to write on my desk by hand without a blotter.

"And by the way," Jim added, "those desks in elementary school? They're made out of maple, not pine."

This pretty much sank Charlie's desk idea as far as I was concerned; maple is rock compared to pine.

So if not white pine, then what? I was pretty much on my own with this one. Jim nominated maple, and showed me a countertop he was building. The wood was almost white, with virtually no discernible grain to it. It made me think of Danish Modern, that kind of sleek blond surface you saw so much of in the sixties—a decidedly unwoody wood, and way too contemporary for this place. What about cherry? It seemed kind of fancy for an outbuilding; I worried it would stand out too much against the workaday fir and plywood. Charlie had said the desk should be of a piece with the other kinds of woods that made up the building, and not too "zippy." So maybe oak? Oak desks were eminently hard and venerable (and not at all zippy), but there's something about the wood that rubs me the wrong way. Oak is almost *too* woody a wood, the wood you see whenever someone wants to say "wood"—by now it's as much a signifier as a thing. It's been simulated so often, in fast-food furniture and hotel case goods, that even the genuine article has begun to look a little fake. Running through the various options, dropping by Jim's shop now and again to look over a sample, I was struck by the amount of cultural freight the various wood species had been made to carry, at least the ones we've seen fit to bring indoors. Selecting a wood for an interior means weighing not only the species' appearance and material qualities, but also the history of its use and whatever architectural fashions have imprinted themselves on it—the mark that Danish Modern has left on maple, say, or Arts and Crafts on oak.

On one of my visits to Jim's, flipping through his racks of furniture stock, I pulled one pale board that wasn't instantly identifiable but which, after I'd raised its grain with a drop of saliva, seemed oddly familiar. I asked him what I was looking at. White ash—of course. I knew it from a hundred garden-tool handles and, back much farther than that, from all those long moments spent in on-deck circles studying the sweeping grain and burnt-in logo on the loin of a Louisville Slugger. I picked up a short length of the ash and realized I had a specific sense memory of its weight, which always takes me slightly by surprise; the wood's paleness prepares your hand for something light, on the order of pine, but ash has a real heft to it, and I knew it to the ounce.

Jim said ash was a fine choice for a desk, even though you didn't see it used that way too often. The wood was hard and wore nicely, yellowing slightly over time, its cream color turning to butter. I asked if I could take a piece of it home.

When I mentioned the idea of ash to Charlie, he was dubious at first, worried it might have the same contemporary associations that maple has, since it was nearly that white. But when I sanded my sample and rubbed a little tung oil into it, the hue of the wood grew warmer. It became apparent that its grain was far more vivid than maple's, with loose, shadowy springwood rings standing out from the intervening regions of dense white summerwood. The pattern and the hue both reminded me of rippled beach sand.

I liked the look of the ash, and also the fact that the wood had no obvious stylistic associations. It made you think of tools before interiors, which I counted a plus, since this was after all a working surface I was making—a tool of a kind. I looked up "ash" in a couple of reference books, and what I read about the tree, which happens to be well represented on my land, gave me a fresh respect for it.

The variety of uses to which white ash has been put is truly impressive, the result of the wood's unusual combination of strength and suppleness: Though hard, it is also pliant enough to take the shapes we give it and to absorb powerful blows without breaking. In addition to baseball bats and a great assortment of tools (including the handles of trowels, hammers, axes, and mallets and the shanks of scythes), I read that ash trees have been recruited over the years for church pews and bowling alleys, the D-handles of spades and shovels and the felloes, or rims, of wooden wheels (the wood obligingly holds its curve when steamed and bent), the oars and keels of small boats, garden and porch furniture, the slats of ladder-back chairs and the seats of swings, pump handles and butter-tub staves, archaic weapons of war including spears, pikes, battle-axes, lances, arrows, and cross-bows (some treaties gave Indians the right to cut ash on any land in America, no matter who owns it), snowshoes, ladder rungs, the axles of horse-drawn vehicles (the first automobiles and airplanes had ash frames), and virtually every piece of sports equipment that is made out of wood, including hockey sticks, javelins, tennis rackets, polo mallets, skis, parallel bars, and the runners on sleds and toboggans.

From the admiring accounts I read, one might conclude that white ash is up there with the opposable thumb in driving the advance of human civilization. It's hard to think of a wood more obliging to man than ash—a tree that supplies the handles for the very axes used to cut down other trees. The reason ash makes such a satisfactory tool handle is that, in addition to its straight grain and supple strength, the wood is so congenial to our hands, wearing smooth with long use and hardly ever splintering. Ash is as useful, necessary, and dependable as work itself, and perhaps for that reason it is no more glamorous. As a tree, I confess I'd always taken the ash pretty much for granted, probably because it grows like a weed around here. But now I was sold. I would make my desk out of the most common tree on the property, the very tree that the window over my desk looked out on.

≡

Ash boards proved somewhat harder to find than ash trees; it seems that most of the board feet cut each year go to makers of tools and sports equipment. Eventually I tracked down a local lumber mill, Berkshire Wood Products, that had a small quantity of native white ash in stock, mixed lengths of five quarter. (Charlie and Joe had both told me I'd be better off with native stock; having already been acclimated to the local air, it would be less likely to check or warp or otherwise surprise.)

Berkshire Wood Products consists of a small collection of ramshackle barns and sheds at the end of a long dirt road in the woods just over the state line in Massachusetts. The place had a distinct old-hippie air about it, with a big vegetable garden out front that was mulched with composted sawdust. Though only a tiny operation, the mill performed every step of the lumber-making process itself, cutting down the tree, milling the logs, kiln-drying the lumber, and dressing the planks to order.

The yardman invited me to select the boards I wanted, pointing to the very top of a three-story-tall rack that filled a large barn. To get to the ash I had to climb a scaffold, moving past handsome rough-sawn slabs of walnut, cherry, white pine, tulip wood, red oak, and yellow birch—most of the important furniture woods of the Northeastern forest. Many of the boards still had their bark, making them look more like tree slices than lumber. I reached the stack of ash and it was gorgeous stuff: eight-foot lengths of creamy white lumber, a handful of the boards set off with elliptical galaxies of nut-brown heartwood stretching out along the grain. Evidently brown heartwood is considered undesirable in ash, because when I expressed particular interest in these boards, the foreman offered to give me a discount.

Only after toting up the total board-foot price did the yardman begin dressing the lumber, much as if I were buying whole fishes I wanted filleted. Working together, he and I ran the best face of each board through the planer several times to remove the rotary scars left by the sawmill, and then used a laser-guided table saw to trim the boards lengthwise, removing the bark and wane and creating the perfectly straight and parallel edges I would need to join the boards cleanly. I realized from his banter that the yardman took me for a carpenter rather than a hobbyist; had I become so conversant in wood that I could actually pass? I loaded the ash in the back of my station wagon and headed home.

Our plan was to glue six of the boards together to make a big, roughly dimensioned plank from which we could then cut out the precise shape of the desk. As we lined up the boards on the floor I decided which ones I liked best and considered where in the finished desktop these should fall. Joe encouraged me to take my time about it: "You're going to have to live with these boards a long time." He clomped away while I ordered and reordered the boards, searching for the most pleasing pattern of grain and figuration. In my parents' living room when I was growing up, there was an English walnut coffee table made by a Japanese woodworker named Nakashima, and the Rorschach-like burls and figures of that surface, which reminded me at various times of clouds and animals and monstrous faces, are printed on my memory as few images from that time are; I can still picture them, vivid and intimate as birthmarks. So I took my sweet time about it, making sure that the most interesting figures fell where, daydreaming at my desk, I would be able to dwell on them.

Once I was satisfied with the arrangement of boards, we painted their edges with wood glue, pressed them up against one another, and then secured the assembly with a pair of clamps, tightening until buttery beads of glue weeped from the seams. In a couple of hours, these six ash boards would be for all purposes one. We gave the assembly overnight to cure and then rough-sanded the surface with Joe's belt sander, smoothing out the joints and removing the dried pearls of glue that had collected along the seams.

Now came the hard and truly harrowing part: cutting the slab to fit the building. Not only did the main section of the desk have to wrap around a corner post and fin wall at either end, but its back edge had to be cut into a toothy pattern matching the two-by-four studs beneath the window. This is how it had to look:

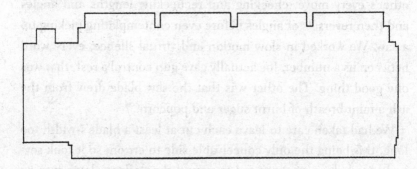

And this is the *platonic* version of the desktop's configuration. I probably don't have to mention that none of what appear in this drawing to be right angles could be exactly that in reality: the cut-away at upper right had to fit the notoriously twisted corner post—the probable cause of our unending headache—and the wing on either side had to be subtly trapezoidal, the right one a couple degrees less subtle than the left. The shape of this desk, in other words, represented the ultimate wages of our original geometrical sin. Less obvious but at least as perilous to our success was the fact that we had to work from the precise mirror image of this design penciled onto the underside of the desktop, since it is an axiom of woodworking that one always cuts from the back side of a finished wood surface in order to prevent the teeth of the saw from marring it.

Any significant error would mean driving back to Berkshire Products and starting all over again.

The day we cut the main section of the desk I remember as the day without small talk; not since my SATs had I put in so many consecutive hours of relentless, single-minded concentration. The subject of this particular test may only have been Euclidean geometry, but there were some hard problems on it calling for the rotation of an imaginary—and radically asymmetrical—object in space, and you weren't allowed to use an eraser, either. So we measured every cut three, sometimes four times, interrogating each other's every move, checking and rechecking lengths and angles and then reversals of angles before even contemplating picking up a saw. We worked in slow motion and virtual silence, every word between us a number. Joe actually gave gun control a rest, that was one good thing. The other was that the saw blade drew from the ash a faint breath of burnt sugar and popcorn.

We had taken care to leave each cut at least a blade's-width too long, this being the only conceivable side to err on, so it took several tries before we managed to pound the desktop down into its tight and tricky pocket, but at last, and with a terrific screeching complaint of wood against wood, it went in. A drive fit. Not quite perfect—there were eighth-inch gaps here and there—but a damned sight closer than I'd ever thought we'd come. A rush of relief is what we mainly felt, our high-fives more exhausted than exultant, but they were no less sweet for that. Though I ran the risk of offending Joe by seeming so surprised, the job we'd done on this desk looked downright professional: here was an actual piece of furniture, and *we'd* made it. "Careful," he cautioned, "a guy could get hurt patting himself on the back like that."

I felt like we'd crossed over a crest of some kind, and from way up here the road ahead sloped down nicely, looking like it might even be smooth.

✓ THE METAPHYSICS OF TRIM

And for a while it was. The following weeks saw steady progress, no disasters. We laid and finished the floor, framed the steps and the daybed, and closed in the rear wall around the daybed with four-inch strips of clear pine. One unseasonably warm March Saturday we moved the operation outdoors, building and hanging the wooden visor over the front window. Charlie had said the cap visor would substantially alter the character of the building, and that it did, relaxing the formality of its classical face, giving it a definite outlook and a personality that seemed much more approachable. "You know, Mike, this building's starting to look like you," Joe announced after the visor went up; he was leaning back in an exaggerated way to fit me and the building into a frame formed with his hands, as if searching for the family resemblance. "Must be the baseball cap," I said.

Joe and I worked methodically and well, achieving an easy collaboration on many of those early spring days. I began to feel less like a helper than a partner, and we traded off tasks depending on our mood rather than on the likelihood of my screwing up something important. I noticed that my finish nails seldom bent anymore (a good thing, too, when you're nailing lengths of clear pine that cost $2 a linear foot), and the circular saw had lost its ability to startle me with short cuts or seize-ups. My grasp of wood behavior was daily growing surer, and I'd internalized all of Joe's sawing saws, which now played in my head like a cautionary mantra: Measure twice cut once, consider all the consequences, remember to count the kerf (the extra eighth of an inch removed by the saw blade itself). As I grew more confident about making field decisions, phone calls to Charlie became infrequent, until one day, concerned about the long spell of radio silence from the job site, Charlie called *me* to see if there was anything we needed. Not that I could think of; we were rolling along. Some days I even got to be the head carpenter in charge, Joe manning the chop saw while I called for lengths of lumber. What it felt like now was a pretty good job, one poised on that fine-point where it is no longer daunting yet still reliably supplies days of novelty and challenge. The hours slipped by, and the end of each workday brought the satisfaction of markable progress and the solidifying conviction that this building was going to get done.

Our happy march down the punch list came to a sudden halt one evening late that spring, when Joe phoned to say he'd broken his hand at work and wouldn't be able to work for three months, possibly longer. He'd been carrying a long stack of two-by-eights when the lumber bumped into something and spasmed, wrenching his hand so far backward that it shattered his metacarpal bone. The doctors had screwed a steel plate to the back of his hand to hold the bone together and warned him not to use it for at least three months. "The only good thing about this I can think of," Joe'd said, bleakly, "is that now I can slip a .45 through an airport metal detector."

I automatically assumed that work on the building would simply halt until Joe's hand was healed. But then I decided that would be just too pathetic. Was I still so dependent on Joe? Of the finish work left to do, I could think of very little that required two men; whatever tools I still needed could be borrowed. I decided that the only self-respecting way to interpret Joe's injury was as a sign it was time to be working on my own.

So the next morning I set to work, solo, if not exactly alone. I started out with easy stuff, cutting lengths of number-two pine on the chop saw and nailing them to the wall beneath my desk, which promised to hide any mistakes in its shadow. But this work went so smoothly that I decided, what the hell, why don't you see if you can't figure out how to trim a window. And this is what I set out to do the following day, working at a pace so excruciatingly deliberate it would undoubtedly have gotten me fired had I not been the boss. But turtling through the work as I did seemed in itself an accomplishment for me, to lay by my ordinary haste and move through a single day as a more patient and deliberate kind of person. I talked to myself the whole time, too, narrating the play-by-play in a rapt murmur I recognized from televised golf.

The syntax of window trim is sternly inflexible, and I reviewed each step of the procedure aloud as if giving instructions to a child, making absolutely sure to cut and nail each trim piece according to the stipulated chronology: skirt first; stool, or sill, on top of that; then a molding up each side; and finally a crown piece butt-jointed across the top of those. By the end of the day I had one perfectly respectable windowsill to my credit, and, between my ears, this gigantic, brain-crowding balloon of pride.

After successfully trimming out another window or two, I found I could get the job done without the chorus of supervisory voices, and my thoughts took their accustomed more speculative turn. The better part of one afternoon I spent trying to decide whether trim was the italics of building, serving to underscore a window or door, or, since trim was also used to bridge dissimilar surfaces and gloss over mistakes, was it instead the transitional phrase—one of those clauses that allows a writer to leap from one idea to another, covering over gaps in logic or narrative with a few cheap words? I concluded trim could be either.

My building had little if any italic trim, and a minimum of transitional or glossing-over trim, certainly fewer pieces of it than there were mistakes in need of forgiveness. As I nailed narrow strips of pine to the window casings, covering the gap between casing and post, I passed the time considering the relationship between trim and human fallibility. To trim, I decided, is human, which probably explains the modernists' contempt for it. Because if we're not using trim to hide our poor craftsmanship, we're using it to proclaim our fine craftsmanship—either way, sloth or pride, trim embodies the most human of failings and thereby spoils the supreme objectivity that modernists strove for.

The machine was supposed to allow us to dispense with trim altogether, by achieving perfect joints beyond the skill of any craftsman. In practice, however, the seamless, untrimmed interior proved as elusive as most other modernist goals: To build to the exacting tolerances seamlessness demanded was prohibitively expensive. The real world holds a powerful brief for trim, it seems. Many modernists also found themselves forced back on the rhetorical possibilities of trim as a way to help "express" the structure of their buildings when simply revealing it wasn't a realistic option. Mies decided to trim the exterior of the Seagram building with purely decorative I-beams when the building code forced him to cake the real ones in layers of unsightly fire retardant.

But even in places where the ideal of trimlessness has been realized, many people have sensed something cold, if not inhuman, in the achievement. Trim seems to speak to our condition, and not only as mistake-makers. Christopher Alexander suggests that its deeper purpose may be to provide a bridge between the simple shapes and proportions of our buildings and a human realm of greater complexity and intimacy. By offering the eye a hierarchy of intermediate-sized shapes, finish trim helps us to make a comfortable perceptual transition from the larger-than-life scale of the whole to the familiar bodily scale of windows and doors, all the way down to the intimate scale of moldings as slender as our fingers. The mathematician and chaos theorist Benoit Mandelbroit makes a similar point when he criticizes modernist architecture for failing to bridge the perceptual distance between its "unnaturally" simple forms and the human scale. Mandelbroit suggests that architectural ornament and trim appeal to us because they offer the eye a complex and continuous hierarchy of form and detail, from the exceedingly fine to the massive, that closely resembles the complex hierarchies we find in nature—in the structure of a tree or a crystal or an animal.

Though plainly not a modernist building, my writing house did exhibit a couple of puzzlingly modernist features: its more or less transparent structure, for example, and its relative lack of trim. But if Alexander and Mandelbroit were right, then the building's own modest scale, as well as the intricate hierarchy of detail that organizes its structure—from the big corner posts to the midsize fin walls down to the exposed three-quarter-inch edge of their plywood faces—meant there was no need for trim to provide transitions from one scale to another or to complexify a shape that would otherwise have seemed "unnaturally" simple. The building was human enough without it.

Nor was Charlie particularly concerned that Joe and I hide our every mistake behind a piece of trim. On the subject of error he liked to quote Ruskin, who had defended the craftsman against the inhumanity of the machine by declaring that "No good work whatever can be perfect, and the demand for perfection is always a sign of a misunderstanding of the ends of art." No misunderstandings here. One time when I asked Charlie whether or not I should install a piece of trim over one particularly unfortunate gap that a mistake of mine had breached between a fin wall and the desk, he argued against it on the grounds trim here would be too finicky. "It's okay for a building like this to have a few holidays," he explained, employing a euphemism for error I'd never heard before; I suppose it has to do with taking the occasional day off from the reigning standards of workmanship, a most human thing to want to do. "Holiday?!" Joe roared when I passed on the comment. "I've got some news for Charlie: This building's a fuckin' Mardi Gras!"

✓ WOOD, FINISHED

One last thing about trim: You don't ordinarily find it in furniture, since it's customary in furniture making to hallow rather than obscure the joinery. I mention this because as I worked at finishing my building's surfaces that summer, I came to see that the whole notion of furniture had more to do with the design and finish of my writing house than I'd ever imagined. I realized that its lack of trim and transparency of structure had less to do with the aesthetic of the Bauhaus than that of the furniture maker, who characteristically strives to make the decorative and the structural one—not by suppressing the decorative, but by elaborating and refining, almost lovingly, his structures. The furniture maker strives to emphasize the beauty of his joints, to highlight the ingenious ways a piece fits together and conveys its weight to the ground, and to bring out the inherent qualities of its materials with his painstakingly hand-worked finishes.

This last labor consumed me for a great many of those Joeless days, as I sanded and oiled all the interior surfaces of my building, a task so vast it made me feel like a mouse trying single-handedly to refinish an armoire. The sanding alone took me over every inch of the interior four separate times: first with the belt sander, to remove the saw marks and lumberyard inks, and thrice more with the palm sander, each time applying a finer and finer grit, until the grain rose up brightly from the muffled surface of blemishes, sanding marks, and pith. Each coat of tung oil required another circumnavigation of the interior, and there were two coats everywhere but on the desk, which received a third and a fourth. Lastly there were the once-overs with steel wool, to remove the tack between coats of oil.

Once I'd acquired the proper frame of mind, or maybe I should say mindlessness, I found finishing to be an exquisite form of drudgery, especially after I'd laid all my power tools aside and taken up the oil cloth. Bringing nothing more than my hands to the task, I slowly rubbed and pressed the wood as if it were muscled flesh, over and over again in a widening spiral of attention. And after a few hours it did begin to feel like some weird interspecies form of massage. The backs of these boards, far from being inanimate, responded to my touch, absorbing the oils and then admitting the light deep into their grain until their complexion completely changed, the wood becoming more essentially and emphatically (and yet at the same time somehow less literally) itself.

Finishing acquainted me with these woods—the species but also the individual boards—in a way nothing we'd done to them until now ever had. Now I knew fir, how the rub of oil elicits its fine salmon hue, and how the small, tight knots in an ordinary two-by-four will fluster the calm sweep of its grain. White pine blushes faintly pink, swirling here and there with nuttier streaks of heart-wood, and as the permanent wetting of the oil brought forward the sweeping grain and figuration of my ash, I could make out beneath the desk's finish what looked like a half-dozen baseball bats flattened out in a kind of Mercator projection. There are boards in this build-ing already as familiar to me as the skin on the back of my hand.

✓ HABITABLE FURNITURE

Two and half years ago, when I mentioned to Charlie that I con-ceived of my building as a piece of furniture, all I had in mind was a particular scale and a tightly ordered, ship-shape layout—cer-tainly not an intricate wooden interior that I would end up sanding and oiling and rubbing every square inch of by hand. But as I went about this work, investing my hours and days in the cultivation of these wood surfaces, I felt like it was indeed a piece of furniture I was finishing and, more, that a piece of furniture was exactly what a "writing house"—a name my building seemed to have grown into—should be. *Why* this should be so I didn't have a clue. Now I think I do.

Blame it on the tung oil fumes, but I began to wonder why it is that studies and libraries are so often finished in wood, in fine stocks and handcrafted panels oiled to resemble furniture. It only made sense that Charlie would have adopted this particular idiom for my writing house, since it is after all a study and a home for books. But where did the convention come from in the first place? I found the outlines of an answer in a couple of histories, and what I read suggested that there might be yet another path along which time finds its way into our buildings, working somewhere beneath the consciousness of architects and builders and inhabitants, but shaping our dreams of place all the same.

The study, it seems, evolved during the Renaissance from a piece of bedroom furniture: the writing desk, escritoire, or secretary, in which a man traditionally kept his ledgers and family documents, usually under lock and key. Personal privacy as we think of it scarcely existed prior to the Renaissance, which is when the wide-open house was first subdivided into specific rooms dedicated to specific purposes; before that time, the locked writing desk was as close to a private space as the house afforded the individual. But as the cultural and political currents of the Renaissance nourished the new humanist conception of self as a distinct individual, there emerged a new desire (at least on the part of those who could afford it) for a place one might go to cultivate this self—for a room of one's own. The man acquired his study, and the woman her boudoir.

Probably the first genuinely private space in the West, the Renaissance study was a small locked compartment that adjoined the master bedroom, a place where no other soul set foot and where the man of the house withdrew to consult his books and papers, manage the household accounts, and write in his diary. Exactly when such rooms became commonplace is hard to date precisely, though under the *OED*'s entry for the word "study," there is a citation from 1430 that would argue for the fifteenth century at the latest: "He passed from chambre to chambre tyle he come yn his secret study where no creature used to come but his self allone."

In Renaissance Italy such a room was called a *studiolo*, which happens to be the same word used to denote a writing desk; at about the same time the French began to use the word *cabinet* to denote a kind of room as well as a locked wooden box. These spaces "grew from an item of furniture to something like furniture in which one lives," I read in Philippe Ariès's five-volume *A History of Private Life*. The new room was essentially the old piece of furniture writ large, an escritoire blown up to habitable dimensions. It was only natural that the new space would preserve the wooden finishes and intricate detailing of its precursor, so that the interiors of a study came to look a lot like the interior of a rolltop desk as seen by, say, a mouse.

I found it uncanny, and somehow almost moving, that this particular bit of history could have inscribed itself on my building without so much as a conscious thought from Charlie or me. But I suppose this is how it usually goes with our buildings: history will have its way with them, whether their architects and builders are historically minded or not. So it happens that every library or study that's ever been finished in wood has as its ancestor the escritoire or *studiolo,* and that the scent of masculinity given off by rooms paneled in dark wood—men's clubs, smoking parlors, speakeasies—has its source in the exclusively male preserve of the study. Here then was yet another sense in which our spaces are wedded ineluctably to our history, to times that, though *we* may have long ago forgotten them, our buildings nonetheless remember.

Perhaps the most famous and influential of all Renaissance studies was the one belonging to Michel de Montaigne. In 1571, at the age of thirty-eight, Montaigne retired from public life—he'd practiced law in Bordeaux, serving for a time as the city's magistrate—to his country estate, where he began to spend the better part of his days in a circular library on the third floor of a tower. Here he read rather aimlessly, jotted down his thoughts now and again, and eventually invented a new literary genre that he decided, with characteristic modesty, to call an "attempt," or essay.

Just what the architectural setting might have had to do with the literary achievement—the new space with the new voice—is impossible to say with certainty. But whenever Montaigne wrote about his study it was in terms that suggested there was a close connection in his mind between the place and the project, a project that has been likened to an exploration of the newly discovered continent of the self.

"When at home I slip off a little more often to my library," he tells us in an essay, "On Three Kinds of Social Intercourse" (being alone with his books is his favorite), "which I like for being a little hard to reach and out of the way." From his tower library, encircled by his books and "three splendid and unhampered views,"

> it is easy for me to oversee my household . . . I am above my gateway and have a view of my garden, my chicken-run, my backyard and most parts of my house. There I can turn over the leaves of this book or that, a bit at a time without order or design. Sometimes my mind wanders off, at others I walk to or fro, noting down or dictating these whims of mine.

It's not hard to find likenesses between the form of the essays and the room in which they took shape. The broad compass of its outlook, the desultory skipping from volume to volume that the bookshelves "curving round me" would have encouraged, the siting of the library such that it allowed Montaigne simultaneously to oversee and withdraw from domestic life—in a great many ways the material facts of Montaigne's study aligned closely with the habits of a mind that ranged widely, that believed the best way to understand Man was by closely examining the circumference of one man's experience (his own), and that relished the minutiae of everyday life. (One of my favorite passages in the essays concerns the pleasures of scratching, a topic I would not have expected literature's *first* essayist to get around to.) The fact that from his desk Montaigne could see both his books and his household—and it was rare at that time for a study even to have a window—mirrors the characteristic movement of his essays, commuting so easily between the evidences of literature and of life. Montaigne's tower also provided him a place from which he could see without being seen, allowing him to withdraw from the world and yet still experience a kind of power over it. "There," he said of his study, "is my throne."

"First we shape our buildings," Winston Churchill famously remarked, "and thereafter our buildings shape us." It may be this kind of reciprocal action that best explains the tie between the Renaissance invention of the study and the age's discovery of the self, an achievement in which Montaigne must be counted a Columbus, and his study the *Santa Maria* on which he set sail. What began as a safe and private place for a man to keep his accounts and genealogies and most closely held secrets gradually evolved into a place one went to cultivate the self, particularly on the page. According to Philippe Ariès, the emergence of a modern sense of privacy and individualism during the Renaissance was closely tied to changes in the literary culture, to the ways that people read and the forms in which they wrote. The discovery of silent reading fostered a more solitary and personal relationship with the book. Then there was the new passion for the writing of diaries, memoirs, and, with Montaigne, personal essays—forms that flourished in the private air of the study, a room that is the very embodiment in wood of the first-person singular.

✓ LIGHT

While I was putting the finishing touches on my own first-person house, a local electrician by the name of Fred Hammond had been busy rigging up its electrical and telephone lines—the last significant hurdle before I could move in. It was one hurdle I decided it would be the better part of valor (Joe's valor, that is: *I'd* never claimed wiring the building ourselves would be a "piece a cake") to leave to a licensed professional. Given my extensive personal history of physical mishap (I've been bitten in the face by a seagull, and once broke my nose falling out of bed), remaining alive and intact for the duration of this project was never something I took for granted, and having avoided serious injury to this point—fingers and toes still coming in at ten and ten—I wasn't about to start fooling around now with volts and amps and alternating current, an alien realm to which my customary haste and reliance on trial and error seemed especially ill-suited.

Fred and his partner Larry happen to be brilliant electricians, but even so my little writing house managed to tax their skill and patience. "This is not normal construction," Fred declared each time he missed a deadline and tossed another cost-estimate out the window. What he meant was that there were no sheetrocked walls or dropped ceilings behind which he could easily run, and hide, his wires. For the same reason, Charlie and I had both resigned ourselves to exposed wires or conduit. But Fred ultimately came up with a much more elegant solution, though it proved to be difficult and time-consuming to execute. The solution involved Fred, the smaller of the two electricians, spending a great many hours stuffed into the eighteen-inch crawl space beneath my building, blindly snaking wires up from there through the closed-in fin walls and bitching lustily the whole time. I give him credit for a masterful wiring job, but if I ever summon the courage to follow Thoreau's example and actually tote up what this house cost me to build, I expect Fred's bill will help push the total into the zone of serious folly. (I'm guessing I spent somewhere in excess of $125 a square foot—for an uninsulated, unplumbed outbuilding, on which half of the construction labor was free.) Fred's complaint—"not normal construction"—could serve very nicely as a legend inscribed over my building's door.

The electricians finished up on a gray and chilly day in November, metallic as only that month can make them, and when Fred and Larry drove off I was elated to have the building to myself again, no more wire snakes, outlet boxes, or complaints to dance around. Now I had light and something that could pass for heat. Joe, whose hand had just about recovered, was due back in a few days to help me hook up the stove; to Charlie's disappointment, I'd opted for kerosene instead of wood, going with a sophisticated little Japanese unit with a microchip that would see to it that the building was toasty by the time I arrived for work in the morning. For the time being, I had a couple of space heaters I could plug in, and so begin to get settled, sort of. All along I'd figured there'd come this one red-letter day when the building would be *finished*, but now I could see it wasn't ever going to be as definitive or ceremonial as all that, no bottle of champagne smashed across the bow. The way things were going, there'd probably be maintenance jobs to start in on before the punch list was completely punched. So I decided I might as well just move in the day after the day Fred and Larry moved out.

I spent what little remained of that afternoon cleaning up inside, sweeping out snips of wire, nails, and sawdust. As I was finishing up, Judith and Isaac paid me a visit, giving me a chance to show off my new lights. Isaac, who'd been an infant when we poured the footings, was a boy now, two and a half years old and able to make the trek out here on his own power. He had brought along a toy tugboat and a copy of *Pat the Bunny*, and before he and Judith headed back to the house, he placed the boat and the book on an empty shelf and took Judith's hand to go. I couldn't tell if Isaac meant the items as a housewarming present or as a way to mark the new space as his own, give him a reason to return.

As darkness came on, I hauled a couple boxes of my books out from the barn and shelved them; book by book, the walls thickened and the room grew warmer. I got in a few trips before nightfall, and on the last, with two crates balanced under my chin, I stopped for a moment at the bottom of the hill to have a look at the writing house, lit up for the first time. It was not a terribly hospitable evening, moonless and blowing fitfully, the leaves recently flown from the trees, and my building seemed a welcome addition to the landscape—this warm-looking, wide-awake envelope of light set down in the middle of the darkening woods. It looked like some kind of a lantern, spilling a woody glow from all four sides. The building seemed to order the shadowy rocks and trees all around it, to wrest a bright space of habitation from the old, indifferent darkness.

I don't want this to sound like some kind of vision, because though my building might have started out that way, a dreamy notion I'd once had, it was more literal than that now. Not just some metaphor or dream, the building I saw in front of me was a new and luminous fact. A new fact in this world, that was plain enough, but also a new fact in my life. That I had dreamt it and then had a hand in making it a fact was more gratifying than I can say, but now I was looking past that, or trying to, wondering, pointlessly perhaps, about how this building I'd helped to shape might come in time to shape me, where the two of us might be headed. Since the day Joe and I got it all closed in the building had reminded me of a wheelhouse, and now that it stood there all lit up on the wide night, a bright windshield gazing out from beneath its visor at some prospect up ahead, it certainly looked to be journeying *some*where.

But now I was dreaming.

I don't think there is a lighted house in the woods anywhere in this world that doesn't hint at a person inside and a story unfolding, and so, it seemed, did mine. As I walked with my crates up the hill toward my cabinet of light, the person that it hinted at was surely recognizable as me, or at least that part of me this room had been built to house. So this was the house for the self that stood a little apart and at an angle, the self that thought a good place to spend the day was between two walls of books in front of a big window overlooking life. The part of me that was willing to wager something worthwhile could come of being alone in the woods with one's thoughts, in a place of one's own, of one's own making. As for the story that this house hinted at, the first part of it you know already, the part about its making; the next wouldn't begin until tomorrow, on move-in day, a morning that from here held the bright promise of all beginnings, of departure, of once upon a time.

Sources

This book is the story of an education, and I had many teachers in addition to Charles Myer and Joe Benney. William Cronon gave me a tour of Frank Lloyd Wright's Wisconsin that was eye-opening. James Evangelisti at Craftsman Woodshops taught me a great deal about wood and woodworking. Everyone at Northwest Lumber was consistently helpful and patient in answering my questions about materials, no matter how ignorant.

And then there were all the books, dozens of which were recommended, and lent to me, by Charlie. Listed below, by chapter, are the principal works referred to in the text, as well as others that influenced my thinking and building.

Chapter 1: A Room of One's Own

Bachelard, Gaston. *The Poetics of Space* (Boston: Beacon Press, 1969).

Thoreau, Henry David. *Walden* (New York: Penguin Classics, 1986).

Walker, Lester. *Tiny Houses* (Woodstock, N.Y.: The Overlook Press, 1987).

Woolf, Virginia. *A Room of One's Own* (New York: Harvest, 1989).

Wright, Frank Lloyd. *The Natural House* (New York: Meridian Books, 1954).

Chapter 2: The Site

For Lewis Mumford's discussion of the siting of houses in America, see *Roots of Contemporary American Architecture* (New York: Dover, 1972).

There's an excellent summary of picturesque landscape theory in *The Villa: Form and Ideology of Country Houses,* by James Ackerman (Princeton: Princeton University Press, 1990). Also useful are William Howard Adams's *Nature Perfected: Gardens Through History* (New York: Abbeville Press, 1991) and *The Poetics of Gardens* by Charles W. Moore, William J. Mitchell, and William Turnbull, Jr. (Cambridge: MIT Press, 1988).

My information on fêng shui comes mainly from *The Living Earth Manual of Feng-Shui* by Stephen Skinner (London: Routledge & Kegan Paul, 1982) and *The Feng-Shui Handbook* by Derek Walters (London: HarperCollins, 1991). I also profited from an interview with William Spear, a fêng shui doctor and the author of *Feng Shui Made Easy* (San Francisco: HarperCollins, 1995).

For further reading on environmental psychology and landscape aesthetics, see:

Appleton, Jay. *The Symbolism of Habitat* (Seattle: University of Washington Press, 1990).

Kellert, Stephen R., and E. O. Wilson. *The Biophilia Hypothesis* (Washington, D.C.: Island Press, 1993).

Tuan, Yi-Fu. *Space and Place: The Perspective of Experience* (Minneapolis: University of Minnesota Press, 1977).

Wilson, E. O. *Biophilia* (Cambridge: Harvard University Press, 1984).

Chapter 3: On Paper

All of Christopher Alexander's books are worth reading, but the best known and most useful to the builder are:

Alexander, Christopher, et al. *A Pattern Language* (New York: Oxford University Press, 1977).

———. *The Timeless Way of Building* (New York: Oxford University Press, 1979).

The awards issue of *Progressive Architecture* I describe is January 1992.

The classic account of the primitive hut myth in architecture is Joseph Rykwert's *On Adam's House in Paradise* (Cambridge: MIT Press, 1981).

Also see the essay on Marc-Antoine Laugier (don't miss the plates) in Anthony Vidler's *The Writing on the Walls: Architectural Theory in the Late Enlightenment* (Princeton: Princeton Architectural Press, 1987) and Laugier's *An Essay on Architecture,* translated by Wolfgang and Anni Hermann (Los Angeles: Hennessey & Ingalls, 1977).

Any exploration of postmodern "literary" architecture must begin with Venturi's two groundbreaking manifestos, *Complexity and Contradiction in Architecture* (New York: The Museum of Modern Art, 1966) and, with Denise Scott Brown and Steven Izenour, *Learning from Las Vegas* (Cambridge: MIT Press, 1972).

For an introduction to the architecture and writing of Peter Eisenman see *Re: Working Eisenman* (London: Academy Editions, 1993). Be sure to read his correspondence with Jacques Derrida. You can also find his writings in almost any issue of *ANY: Architecture New York,* a bimonthly broadsheet journal published out of his office and edited by his wife.

Sophisticated critiques of the "linguistic turn" in architecture are hard to come by. I found these three persuasive and useful:

Benedikt, Michael. *Deconstructing the Kimbell: An Essay on Meaning and Architecture* (New York: SITES/Lumen Books, 1991).
———. *For an Architecture of Reality* (New York: Lumen Books, 1987).
Shepheard, Paul. *What Is Architecture? An Essay on Landscapes, Buildings, and Machines* (Cambridge: MIT Press, 1994).

Chapter 4: Footings

The best writing about the importance of the ground, and the horizontal, in American architecture is by the architectural historian Vincent Scully. See *American Architecture and Urbanism* (New York: Praeger Publishers, 1969); *Architecture: The Natural and the Manmade* (New York: St. Martin's Press, 1991); and *The Shingle Style and the Stick Style* (New Haven: Yale University Press, 1955). See also the discussion of *Walden* and Fallingwater in *Forests: The Shadow of Civilization* by Robert Pogue Harrison (Chicago: University of Chicago Press, 1992).

Wright's own comments on the ground are drawn from *The Natural House* (op. cit., Chapter 1) and *The Future of Architecture* (New York: Horizon Press, 1953).

There's a useful discussion of foundations and wood in *A Good House* by Richard Manning (New York: Grove Press, 1993) and a great riff on concrete by Peter Schjeldahl, "Hard Truths About Concrete," in the October 1993 *Harper's Magazine*. Mark Wigley offers a close reading of architectural metaphors in Western philosophy in *The Architecture of Deconstruction: Derrida's Haunt* (Cambridge: MIT Press, 1993).

Chapter 5: Framing

Frank Lloyd Wright's discussion of the origins of architecture and the role of trees is in *The Future of Architecture* (op. cit., Chapter 4).

My account of the origins of balloon framing and its environmental significance draws on William Cronon's *Nature's Metropolis: Chicago and the Great West* (New York: W. W. Norton, 1991). For the social history of timber framing in America (including the evergreen ritual) I relied on John Stilgoe's *Common Landscape of America, 1580–1845* (New Haven: Yale University Press, 1982). Everyone who writes on the social meaning of building methods in America owes a large debt to the essays of the late J. B. Jackson. See *The Necessity for Ruins* (Amherst: The University of Massachusetts, 1980) and *Discovering the Vernacular Landscape* (New Haven: Yale University Press, 1984).

Hannah Arendt's account of *homo faber,* and the distinctions between work and labor, appear in *The Human Condition* (New York: Doubleday, 1959).

For a wonderful discussion of shame and sacrifice rituals, see Frederick Turner's *The Culture of Hope* (New York: Free Press, 1995).

Chapter 6: The Roof

As much of this chapter took place in the library as up on the roof. Here's a partial list of my readings on roofness and architectural theory:

Alexander, Christopher, and Peter Eisenman. "Contrasting Concepts of Harmony: A Debate" in *Lotus International* (1983). This is the text of a fascinating, and heated, public debate held at the Harvard Graduate School of Design.

Argyros, Alexander J. *A Blessed Rage for Order: Deconstruction, Evolution, and Chaos* (Ann Arbor: University of Michigan Press, 1991).

Benedikt, Michael. *Deconstructing the Kimbell* and *For an Architecture of Reality* (op. cit., Chapter 3).

———, ed. "Buildings and Reality: Architecture in the Age of Information," a special issue of *Center: A Journal for Architecture in America* (New York: Rizzoli, 1988).

Bloomer, Kent C., and Charles W. Moore. *Body, Memory, and Architecture* (New Haven: Yale University Press, 1977).

Cronon, William. "Inconstant Unity: The Passion of Frank Lloyd Wright," in *Frank Lloyd Wright: Architect*, Terence Riley, ed. (New York: The Museum of Modern Art, 1994).

Crowe, Norman. *Nature and the Idea of a Man-Made World* (Cambridge: MIT Press, 1995).

Eisenman, Peter. *Re: Working Eisenman* (op. cit., Chapter 3).

Ford, Edward R. *The Details of Modern Architecture* (Cambridge: MIT Press, 1990).

———. *The Details of Modern Architecture*, Vol. 2 (Cambridge: MIT Press, 1996).

Frampton, Kenneth. *Studies in Tectonic Culture: The Poetics of Construction in Nineteenth and Twentieth Century Architecture* (Cambridge: MIT Press, 1995).

Frank, Suzanne. *Peter Eisenman's House VI: The Client's Response* (New York: Whitney Library of Design, 1994).

Hildebrand, Grant. *The Wright Space: Pattern and Meaning in Frank Lloyd Wright's Houses* (Seattle: University of Washington Press, 1991).

Jackson, J. B. *Landscapes* (Amherst: University of Massachusetts Press, 1970). His description of Grand Central Station is on page 83.

Kahn, Louis. *Between Silence and Light: Spirit in the Architecture of Louis I. Kahn* (Boulder: Shambhala, 1979).

Lyndon, Donlyn, and Charles W. Moore. *Chambers for a Memory Palace* (Cambridge: MIT Press, 1994).

Norberg-Schultz, Christian. *Architecture: Meaning and Place* (New York: Rizzoli, 1988).

———. *Genius Loci: Toward a Phenomenology of Architecture* (New York: Rizzoli, 1980).

———. *New World Architecture* (New York: The Architectural League of New York, 1988).

Rasmussen, Steen Eiler. *Experiencing Architecture* (Cambridge: MIT Press, 1959).

Rudofsky, Bernard. *Architecture Without Architects* (Albuquerque: University of New Mexico Press, 1987).

Rykwert, Joseph. *On Adam's House in Paradise* (op. cit., Chapter 3).

Schwartz, Frederic, ed. *Mother's House: The Evolution of Vanna Venturi's House in Chestnut Hill* (New York: Rizzoli, 1992).

Scully, Vincent. *The Shingle Style Today, or The Historian's Revenge* (New York: George Braziller, 1974). His discussion of the taboo against pitched roofs appears on page 15.

Shepheard, Paul. *What Is Architecture?* (op. cit., Chapter 3).

Venturi, Robert. *Complexity and Contradiction in Architecture* and *Learning from Las Vegas* (op. cit., Chapter 3).

———. *Iconography and Electronics: Upon a Generic Architecture* (Cambridge: MIT Press, 1996).

Vidler, Anthony. *The Writing of the Walls* (op. cit., Chapter 3).

———. *The Architectural Uncanny* (Cambridge: MIT Press, 1992).

Vitruvius. *The Ten Books of Architecture*, translated by Morris Hicky Morgan (New York: Dover, 1960). His description of architectural evolution appears in "Origin of the Dwelling House," pages 38–41.

Wigley, Mark. *The Architecture of Deconstruction: Derrida's Haunt* (op. cit., Chapter 4).

See also *The Cedar Shake and Shingle Bureau Design and Application Manual* (Farmingdale, New York).

Chapter 7: Windows

On the history of the idea of transparency in the West, I relied on Richard Sennett's *The Conscience of the Eye: The Design and Social Life of Cities* (New York: W. W. Norton, 1990). Also helpful on the subject of glass in architecture were Robert Hughes, in his terrific chapter on modern architecture in *The Shock of the New* (New York: Alfred A. Knopf, 1980), and Reyner Banham's *The Architecture of the Well-Tempered Environment* (London: The Architectural Press, 1969). See also John Berger's *Ways of Seeing* (London: BBC & Penguin, 1972) and Norman Bryson's *Vision and Painting: The Logic of the Gaze* (New Haven: Yale University Press, 1972).

By far the most provocative article I've read on windows is Neil Levine's "Questioning the View: Seaside's Critique of the Gaze of Modern Architecture" in *Seaside: Making a Town in America,* edited by David Mohney and Keller Easterling (Princeton: Princeton Architectural Press, 1991). See also the chapter on transparency in Vidler's *The Architectural Uncanny* (op. cit., Chapter 6) and, though I don't claim to understand all of it, Colin Rowe's seminal essay (with Robert Slutzky) "Transparency: Literal and Phenomenal" in *The Mathematics of the Ideal Villa and Other Essays* (Cambridge: MIT Press, 1976).

Chapter 8: Finish Work

On the place of time in architecture, see:

Brand, Stewart. *How Buildings Learn* (New York: Viking, 1994).

Jackson, J. B. *A Sense of Place, a Sense of Time* (New Haven: Yale University Press, 1994).

Johnson, Philip. "Whence and Whither: The Processional Element in Architecture," in David Whitney and Jeffrey Kipnis, eds. *Philip Johnson: The Glass House* (New York: Pantheon Books, 1993).

Lynch, Kevin. *What Time Is the Place?* (Cambridge: MIT Press, 1972).

Mostafavi, Mohsen, and David Leatherbarrow. *On Weathering* (Cambridge: MIT Press, 1993).

My principal sources on trees and woods were Herbert L. Edlin's *What Wood Is That? A Manual of Wood Identification* (New York: Viking Press, 1969) and Donald Culross Peattie's *A Natural History of Trees of Eastern and Central North America* (Boston: Houghton Mifflin, 1966).

Benoit Mandelbrot's ideas about architectural ornament are discussed briefly in James Gleick's *Chaos: Making a New Science* (New York: Viking, 1987).

On the history of the study and the rise of the modern individual the key work is *A History of Private Life,* edited by Philippe Ariès and Georges Duby. See Volume III, *Passions of the Renaissance,* especially Ariès's introduction, as well as "The Refuges of Intimacy" by Orest Ranum, and "The Practical Impact of Writing" by Roger Chartier. See also John Lukacs's essay "The Bourgeois Interior" in *The American Scholar* (Vol. 39, No. 4, Autumn 1970) and Mark Wigley's essay "Untitled: The Housing of Gender" in *Sexuality and Space,* edited by Beatriz Colomina (Princeton: Princeton Architectural Press, 1992). Montaigne's description of his study appears in "On Three Kinds of Social Intercourse" in Book III of *Michel de Montaigne: The Complete Essays,* translated by M. A. Screech (New York: Penguin, 1987).

Index

Addison, Joseph, 33
Alberti, Leon Battista, 87
Alexander, Christopher:
  on control, 276
  on enclosure vs. freedom, 97
  on memory in a house, 78, 274
  on patterns, 74–78, 215
  on trim, 290, 291
  on windows, 75, 76–77, 216–17, 261
appearances, worldly, 55–56, 70
Appleton, Jay, 49, 50
architects:
  authority of, 163–64, 165
  and builders, 26, 113–14, 127,
    137–38, 161–65, 179, 223–31,
    245, 278, 279
  and compromise, 130, 231
  and control, 276–77
  and detail, 11, 88–89, 129, 190
  and materials, 199–200
  and orderliness, 11, 12
  and originality, 230
  see also specific architects
Architecture (magazine), 65n
architecture:
  art of, 87, 276
  centrifugal houses, 20–21, 22
  and construction, 87, 150, 203
  and culture, 204, 207, 216,
    218–19, 250
  deconstructivist, 67–69, 155,
    193–97

evolution of, 215–17
Fibonacci Series in, 62
fundamental assumptions of, 193
glass in, 20–21, 184, 248–57
Golden Section in, 62, 79–80, 92,
    112
"magazine," 204
modernist, see modernism
and nature, 79, 87–88, 125,
    135–36, 177, 196, 197, 199,
    207, 216
and nostalgia, 192
origins of, 87, 135
post-and-beam vs. balloon framing
    in, 144, 145–50
postmodernist, 69, 185–88,
    189–91, 192, 244, 245
primitive hut in, 20, 86–88, 135,
    177, 196, 216
pure Idea in, 197
reading the language of, 67,
    187–88, 192–93, 200, 206,
    214–15, 217
and relationship of buildings to
    land, 21, 99–102, 103, 104, 106,
    108, 125
and time, 271–75
unreality in, 67–69, 155, 193–97
vernacular, 244–45
and words, 67–70, 74–78, 187, 215
Arendt, Hannah, 55, 70, 165
Ariès, Philippe, 8, 295, 297

Aristotle, 213
Art in America, 195
Arts and Crafts movement, 237–38,
    240, 244, 245, 258, 281
attic, and pitched roof, 184
authority:
    of architects, 163–64, 165
    of builders, 165
    of columns, 214–15, 216
    of foundations, 120–25, 156

Bachelard, Gaston, 6–7, 8, 18, 19, 21,
    74, 184
back-to-the-land movement, 244–45
balloon framing, 136, 145–52
    early use of, 150–52
    and impermanence, 151–52
    vs. post-and-beam, 144, 145–50
Benjamin, Walter, 250
Benney, Joe, 109–15, 131
    and finish work, 267–71, 277,
        283–88, 297, 299
    and footings, 111–20, 122–23,
        125–27, 129
    and framing, 136–40, 143–46,
        154–58, 161–72
    injury of, 154, 288
    and interior space, 210–11
    and politics, 225–27, 286
    and roof, 178–79, 181, 188–89,
        198, 200, 207–8, 220
    and windows, 223–24, 227–30,
        257–59
Bergman, Jules, 18
Berkshire Wood Products, 283–84
Biophilia (Wilson), 49
birdhouse, Charlie's design for, 205–7
bird's mouth, 178
bookshelves, 93, 299
Brand, Stewart, 274
Brooklyn Bridge, 100
Brown, Capability, 35, 47
builders:
    and architects, 26, 113–14, 127,
        137–38, 161–65, 179, 223–31,
        245, 278, 279
    authority of, 165
    and standard dimensions, 228–30
building (verb), *see* construction
building code, 80, 115, 125

building permit, 80, 115–17
buildings:
    "buildingness" of, 74
    as gardens, 221
    history of, 295
    imagery and structure of, 187, 202,
        204–7
    relationship of land and, 21,
        99–102, 103, 104, 106, 108, 125
    ruins of, 123–24
    see also architecture; *specific buildings*

carpenters, *see* builders
carpentry:
    building windows, 239–45
    craft of, 137, 240–45, 269, 289–90
    cutting rafters, 178
    finish work of, 267–75, 277–97
    joinery, 136–38, 144, 145, 150, 291
    kerf in, 287
    "measure twice, cut once" in, 140,
        287
    mortising in, 141, 144, 153, 240
    toe-nailing in, 147
    tools of, 138–39, 140–42, 144,
        146, 240–41
    trueness in, 155
    and wood vs. steel, 137
Cartesian grid, 32, 52, 213
cathedral ceiling, 180
cedar shingles, 197–99, 278
centrifugal houses, 22
    vs. centripetal attractors, 19
    of Wright, 20–21
chi:
    in fêng shui, 43–47, 48, 209
    of interior space, 210
    and water, 45–46, 47
    and windows, 236
Churchill, Winston, 297
column, authority of, 214–15, 216
Common Landscape of America
    (Stilgoe), 149
communication:
    electronic, 218–20
    of experience, 217
    meaning as function of, 206–7
    vs. space, 203–4
compromise, 122–24, 130–31, 231,
    236

concrete, 117–20
Conscience of the Eye, The (Sennett), 247
construction:
  and architecture, 87, 150, 203
  balloon framing in, 136, 145–52
  do-it-yourself, 5, 21–29
  and gardening, 25
  mortise and tenon, 136–38, 141, 144, 153, 240
  physical labor vs. abstraction of, 25
  post-and-beam, 86, 136–38, 143–50
  reading about vs. doing, 56–57, 71
  of stone, 151
  and writing, 26
Le Corbusier:
  architecture defined by, 230
  on defying time and decay, 125, 272
  on First Shelter, 87
  on geometry, 112
  and Golden Section, 79
  and modernism, 102, 106, 112, 183, 272–73
corner posts, *see* posts, corner
Cornwall rock, 126
Crane, Hart, 100
Crusoe, Robinson, 87
culture:
  and architecture, 204, 207, 216, 218–19, 250
  and landscape, 25

Darwin, Charles, 49, 76
daydreaming, 7–8, 14–15
deconstruction, 67–69, 155, 193–97
dentils, 190–91
Derrida, Jacques, 54, 121, 193
Descartes, René, 121
design, 90–98
  activity vs., 274–77
  architect and, *see* Myer, Charles R.
  of finish work, 273
  for footings, 103–4, 107
  and mental images, 57–60, 96–97
  preliminary drawings of, 78–90
  and site, 91, 92
  and space, 97
  and walls, 63–64, 97
  watching process of, 60, 71, 78–85

desk, 278–87
  evolution of, 294
  preparation of, 284–86
  shape of, 285–86
  wood for, 279–84
destination:
  need for, 13
  room of one's own as, 14
  welcome to, 299–300
do-it-yourself construction, 21–29
Don (tall friend), 167, 169–70
doorness, 72–73
Douglas fir, 133–36, 143, 147, 158, 175, 214, 278
drawing, 71–90
  as canonical, 137–38
  and experience, 73
  and geometry, 84
  preliminary, 78–90
  and reality, 83–85, 112
  tower scheme, 82–85, 86
dream:
  of enclosure vs. freedom, 97
  of escape, 3–4, 6
  "hut," 19, 27–28, 42, 43
  rationale for, 6
  as shaped by site, 34, 43, 57
  space in which to, 7–8

Eisen, Charles, 88
Eisenman, Peter, 60, 202–3, 204, 216
  on deconstruction, 68–69, 193
  designs by, 66–68
  House VI by, 193–97, 204, 215
electric wiring, 297–99
electronic communication, 218–20
Emerson, Ralph Waldo, 21, 248
Enlightenment, and nature, 247
entrance, 72–73, 77–78
environmentalism, and landscape, 256
Escher, M. C., 66
essays, of Montaigne, 295–97
Euclidian geometry, 52, 149, 155, 213, 286
Evangelisti, Jim:
  and craftsmanship, 244, 245
  and windows, 234–35, 237, 239–45, 246, 257–58
  and writing desk, 278–81
evolution, 206–7, 215–17

Fallingwater, 102, 181, 201*n*
fêng shui, 32, 43–48
  and astrology, 44
  chi in, 43–48
  and gardens, 44
  geomancer of, 45, 46, 47
  riding the dragon in, 46–47
Fibonacci Series, 62
finish work, 267–301
  bookshelves, 299
  built-ins, 273, 276–77, 291–93
  design of, 273
  drudgery of, 292–93
  inhabitants and, 275–78
  light, 297–301
  margin of error in, 268–69
  sanding, 292
  time and place for, 271–75
  trim, 269–70, 272, 277, 287–91
  and untrimmed interior, 290
  wood, finished, 291–97
  writing desk, 278–87, 294
First Shelter, 87
flat vs. pitched roof, 183–88, 189,
    201–2, 245
Flaubert, Gustave, 276
follies, 33
footings, 99–131
  and building permit, 115, 117
  and compromise, 122–24, 130–31
  corner posts, 125–26, 127–29
  design for, 103–4, 107
  dry wall, 101
  elevations of, 139
  and ground, 108
  holes for, 110–11
  pouring of, 117–20
  in rock, 90, 95, 103–4, 107–15,
    125–30
foundationalism, 121
foundations:
  authority and prestige of, 120–25,
    156
  initial ideas about, 86–87
  and metaphysics, 121–22
  out of square, 156–57
  and relationship of buildings to
    land, 99–102, 125
  see also footings

framing, 132–75
  balloon, 136, 144, 145–50
  and geometry, 147, 149
  and interior, 208–11
  joinery and, 136–38
  out of square, 154–57, 160–61,
    167
  post-and-beam, 136–38, 143–44
  raising the ridge pole, 165–71
  and space, 145, 150
  timber, 144, 150, 151–53, 154, 165
  top plate of, 158–61
  treeness of, 144–45
Frank, Dick and Suzanne, 194–97
furniture, 291–97

gabled roof, 183–88, 189, 201–2, 245
gardens:
  buildings as, 221
  and fêng shui, 44
  natural look of, 33
  shaping landscape in, 25, 32–33,
    40, 42
  symbolism of, 221
Gehry, Frank, 66
geometry, 112, 155, 178–79, 220
  and compromise, 122–23
  and framing, 147, 149
  and initial drawings, 84
  and modernism, 184
  and space, 32, 52, 213
  and writing desk, 286
glass houses, 20–21, 184, 248–57
glazing, 242, 253–57, 258
Goethe, Johann Wolfgang von, 66
Golden Section, 62, 79–80, 92, 112
Grand Central Station, 212–13, 214,
    215, 274
gravity, 202–3, 204–7
Greene and Greene, 235, 237–39,
    242, 243, 244, 245
ground, *see* land

Hammond, Fred, 297–298
Heidegger, Martin, 121
Hejduk, John, 204
Here vs. There, 104–7, 124, 204, 221
historic preservation, 244
History of Private Life, A (Ariès), 295

houseness, 16–19
  escape in, 18–19
  shelter in, 16–18, 202–7
houses, *see* architecture; buildings;
  specific houses; writing hut
House VI, 193–97, 204, 215
How Buildings Learn (Brand), 274
Human Condition, The (Arendt), 165
"hut dream," 19, 27–28, 42, 43; *see
  also* primitive hut image

ice dams, 200–201
Idea, pure, 197
information overload, 53–54
interior space, 208–14
  landscape and, 209
  selecting wood for, 281
  and trim, 269–70, 272, 277,
    287–91
  use of, 273, 277, 290
  see also finish work

Jackson, J. B., 151, 152, 212–13, 274
Jefferson, Thomas, 105–6, 151
  Cartesian grid of, 32, 52
  honeymoon cottage of, 22
  and Monticello, 58, 100, 106, 248
Jenks, Bill, 115–17, 125, 129, 130
Johnson, Philip, 106, 194, 248, 249,
  253
joinery, 136–38, 144, 145, 150, 291
joist hanger, 136–38

Kahn, Lloyd, 202
Kahn, Louis, 199
Kant, Immanuel, 121
Kent, William, 35
kerf, 287
kerosene stove, 299
Knerr, Don, 90

land:
  and foundation, 99–102, 125; *see
    also* footings
  freezing and thawing of, 108–9
  and horizontal expansiveness,
    100–101
  relationship of buildings and, 21,
    99–102, 103, 104, 106, 108, 125

and Vietnam Veterans Memorial,
  100, 124
walking, 36–40
yin and yang, 45
landscape:
  aesthetic of, 33, 40
  chi of, 44
  and culture, 25
  curved paths in, 34–35
  and environmentalism, 256
  and fêng shui, 46
  and house, 151, 152–53, 300
  and interior space, 209
  psychological experience of, 33, 97
  self as center of, 38–39
  shaping of, 25, 32–35, 40, 42
  and survival, 49–51
  and trees, 153
  vs. wider world, 104–7
  and windows, 236, 247, 248, 252,
    254–56
Laugier, Marc-Antoine, 87, 88, 104
Learning from Las Vegas (Venturi),
  69–70, 186, 218–19
light, 297–301
  electric wiring for, 297–99
  and unfolding stories, 300–301
  and welcome, 299–300
  windows as source of, 75, 77, 246,
    248, 262
literature, primitive hut in, 87
*Living Earth Manual of Feng-Shui,
  The* (Skinner), 44
Loos, Adolph, 270
Louisville Sluggers, 281
Low house, Bristol RI, 188
Lynch, Kevin, 80

McKim, Mead, and White, 188
McLuhan, Marshall, 54
magazine architecture, 204
Mandelbroit, Benoit, 290–91
materials, honoring, 199–200,
  249–50, 272, 278
"measure twice, cut once," 140, 287
media:
  electronic, 218–20
  and magazine architecture, 204
memory, in each house, 78, 274

metaphysics, 121–22
Mies van der Rohe, Ludwig, 248, 276, 290
mistakes, 58, 291
modernism:
  and corporate America, 192
  Here vs. There in, 106
  and interior design, 270, 272, 273–74, 290
  vs. postmodernism, 245
  psychological hygiene of, 184
  and technology, 256–57
  and time, 272, 274
  and transparency, 249, 253–57, 264
Montaigne, Michel de, 295–97
Monticello, 58, 100, 106, 248
Moore, Charles, 60, 245
mortise and tenon, 136–38, 141, 144, 153, 240
Mumford, Lewis, 31, 32, 67
muntins, 245–53, 256
Myer, Charles R., 8–14
  album from, 61–65, 70, 71–74, 75, 78, 81, 97
  birdhouse designed by, 205–7
  on custom work, 229–30, 265–66, 278
  design by, 90–98, 189–90, 199, 224, 269–70
  and finish work, 269–71, 275–77, 287–88, 291, 293, 298–99
  and footings, 103–4, 107, 108, 110–15, 117, 125–30
  and framing, 136–39, 145, 158–65
  house renovated by, 9–10, 13, 27
  influences on, 60–61, 244–45
  letter to, 57–60, 96–97
  physical appearance of, 11
  preliminary drawings by, 78–90
  and roof, 178–82, 190–91, 197, 199–200, 220
  and site selection, 28–29, 38, 41, 42, 51
  and windows, 224–25, 227–36, 260–61, 263, 265–66
  and writing desk, 278–81, 283
  and writing hut idea, 13–14, 28–29

Nakashima, George, 284
Natural House, The (Wright), 101

nature:
  and architecture, 79, 87–88, 125, 135–36, 177, 196, 197, 199, 207, 216
  birdhouse in, 205–7
  and Enlightenment, 247
  evolution in, 206–7, 215–17
  forest in, 135–36
  in gardens, 25, 33
  Golden Section in, 79
  man's relationship to, 178*n*, 256–57, 264–65
  and place, 104, 106
  rain and gravity, 202–3, 204–7
  reclamation by, 123–25, 272
  refuge from, 18, 20, 21, 97, 246
  and sacrifice, 173
  transparency to, 20, 21, 246–49, 255–57, 263–66
Nonquit, Cape Cod, 81–82

objectivity, 246
orientation, of site, 31–32, 42–43, 45, 111

Palladio, Andrea, 100
paths, curved, 34–35
Pattern Language, A (Alexander), 74–78
perfection, opacity of, 258, 291
perspective:
  and site selection, 4, 35–36, 37, 43
  and windows, 10, 12–13, 27–28, 33, 246, 260–61, 263–65
Peter Eisenman's House VI: The Client's Response (Frank), 194
picture windows, 251, 252, 254–56
pitched vs. flat roof, 183–88, 189, 201–2, 245
placeness, 38–39, 104, 106, 274–75
Plato, 56
Pliny, 118
Poetics of Space, The (Bachelard), 7, 19, 74, 184
Pollan, Isaac, 22, 92, 158, 299
Pollan, Judith, 42
  and construction project, 27
  pregnancy of, 5, 40, 92
  and site selection, 39, 40, 41
  space of, 6, 27

Pollan, Lori, 18
Pope, Alexander, 33
porches, framing of, 264
Portland cement, 118, 119
post-and-beam construction, 86,
    136–38, 143–50
  vs. balloon framing, 144, 145–50
  and "treeness," 144
postmodernism, 189–91, 244
  evolution of, 192
  vs. modernism, 245
  and semiotics, 69
  Vanna Venturi house, 185–88, 189
posts, corner:
  anchors for, 127–29
  cutting of, 139
  detail of, 88–90, 94
  footings for, 90, 127–30
  minisills for, 129–30
  mortises and, 153
  out of square, 154–57
  "postness" of, 89
  pressure-treated, 125–26, 129–30
  space defined by, 95
  as trees, 132–36, 156
preservation, historic, 244
primitive hut image:
  architecture and, 20, 86–88, 135,
      177, 196, 216
  and author's writing hut, 86–88, 95,
      96, 219
  in literature, 87
  roof in, 177
  and trees, 135–36
Progressive Architecture, 61, 64,
    65–71, 183, 188

rafters, cutting, 178
Rand, Ayn, 14, 164
reading:
  architectural language, 67, 187–88,
      192–93, 200, 206, 214–15, 217
  vs. doing, 55–57, 71
  words on paper, 54–56, 70
refuge, *see* shelter
Renaissance:
  privacy in, 294–97
  self and space in, 8
Repton, Humphry, 47
Ricketson, Daniel, 23

ridge pole, raising of, 165–71
rock:
  Cornwall, 126
  and design, 91, 92
  footings in, 90, 95, 103–4, 107–15,
      125–30
roof, 73, 176–222
  bird's mouth of, 178
  capping of, 207
  and cathedral ceiling, 180
  cutting rafters for, 178
  dentils and, 190–91
  and figurative language, 182–83
  gabled, 183–88, 189, 201–2, 245
  and ice dams, 200–201
  leaky, 197, 201, 202–3, 236
  pitched vs. flat, 183–88, 189,
      201–2, 245
  of primitive hut, 177
  as shelter, 180, 201, 216, 220–22
  shingling, 188–89, 190, 197–99,
      207
  starting from zero, 183–86
  steepness of pitch of, 189,
      200–201, 212
  straps on, 179–80, 190–91, 200
  vernacular, 201
Room of One's Own, A (Woolf), 7–8
Rorty, Richard, 54
Rousseau, Jean-Jacques, 247
Ruskin, John, 291

sacrifice, in topping-out ceremony,
    171–75
St. Mary's Catholic Church, Chicago,
    150
Saussure, Ferdinand de, 186
savanna, and survival, 49
Scheerbart, Paul, 249–50
Scully, Vincent, 184, 185, 271
semiotics, semiology, 69, 186, 188
Sennett, Richard, 247, 251
Shaw, George Bernard, 22, 23
shelter:
  centrifugal, 20–21, 22
  First, 87
  first person singular, 23
  and houseness, 16–18, 202–7
  house within house, 18–19, 21
  roof as, 180, 201, 216, 220–22

shelter (cont.):
  and survival, 49–51
  tiny, 22–23
  under siege, 16–18
  and weather, 18, 20, 21, 97
shingles, 197–99, 278
Shingle Style Today, The (Scully), 184
simplification, fantasy of, 4
site, 30–52
  betweenness of, 42
  chi of, 43–47, 209
  and design, 91, 92
  dream shaped by, 34, 43, 57
  everyplace as, 36
  and fêng shui, 32, 43–48
  flow of space at, 91
  and Here vs. There, 104–7
  hospitality of, 32
  and landscape, 32–35, 40
  orientation of, 31–32, 42–43, 45,
    111
  and perspective, 4, 35–36, 37, 43
  as "pleasing prospect," 33–34, 41,
    50, 52
  prospect and refuge of, 49–51, 97,
    209, 213
  and reality, 28–29
  selecting, 30–43
  sense of place in, 274–75
  and topography, 32
  walking the land, 36–40
  as Wilderness, 12–13
Skinner, Stephen, 44
solitude, place of, 3–4, 8
sonotubes, 119
space:
  American sense of, 19–21
  body's experience of, 52, 74,
    210–16
  Cartesian grid of, 32, 52, 213
  communication vs., 203–4
  consensual, 21
  corner posts and, 95
  for daydreaming, 7–8
  and design, 97
  framing and, 145, 150
  of Grand Central Station, 212–13,
    214, 215, 274
  habitation of, 273–75

  horizontal expansiveness in,
    100–101
  interior, 208–14
  of my own, 5–6, 23, 28
  and nonexistent walls, 73
  Renaissance idea of, 8
  sense of place in, 19, 274–75
  at site, 91
  tropisms of, 19, 213
  vertical or tower view of, 19, 82–85,
    86
  and windows, 236, 249
  within space, 18–19, 92
  to work in, 6
steel:
  structural, 250
  vs. wood, 137
Stevens, Wallace, 38, 39, 52
Stickley, Gustav, 240
Stilgoe, John, 149, 171
stone building, 151
stove, kerosene, 299
straps, 179–80, 190–91, 200
structuralists, 186
structure, building as, 187, 202,
    204–7
study, evolution of, 294–97
survival, 49–51
symbolism, and survival, 207
Symbolism of Habitat, The (Appleton),
    50

Tanguay, Tude, 231, 234, 235
television, 218–19
territory:
  and chaos vs. civilization, 17
  and houseness, 16–18
Thoreau, Henry David, 17, 23, 150
  and foundations, 120, 122
  and primitive hut image, 87, 219
  on roofs, 221–22
  on site selection, 36, 37, 38–39, 42,
    43
  at Walden, 19–20, 21, 24, 54, 142,
    222, 264
  and windows, 248–49, 265
time, and architecture, 271–75
Timeless Way of Building, The (Alexan-
    der), 76, 274

Tiny Houses (Walker), 22–23, 61
toe-nailing, 147
tools:
  chain saw, 138–39, 140–41
  chisel, 140–42, 144
  hammer, 146
  machine, 240–41
  rotary hammer, 126
topping-out ceremony, 171–75
top plate, 158–61
tourism, and landscape, 256
tower view, 19, 82–85, 86
transparency:
  and glass houses, 20–21, 184,
    248–57
  virtual, 251–52
  and windows, 246–57, 263–66
tree house, 15–18
trees:
  vs. dimension lumber, 134–35, 147
  intimacy with, 142–43
  landscape and, 153
  large timbers, 135–36, 153
  lumber as abstraction of, 133,
    134–35
  and primitive hut, 135–36
  in topping-out ceremony, 171–75
  "treeness" of, 144–45, 175
  use of, 132–36, 150, 152, 156, 169,
    174
trim, 269–70, 272, 277, 287–91
Turner, Frederick, 173

Venturi, Robert, 193*n*, 202–3, 204
  on electronic communication,
    218–19
  gabled roof by, 185–86, 187
  Learning from Las Vegas by, 69–70,
    186, 218–19
  and postmodernism, 69, 95, 185,
    187–88, 189–91, 192
  and semiotics, 69–70, 186, 188
Venturi, Vanna, house for, 185–88,
    246
Vietnam Veterans Memorial, Washing-
    ton DC, 100, 124
Vitruvius, 177, 178*n*
  on evolution of architecture,
    215–17

and First Shelter, 87
  on site orientation, 31–32, 45
  Vitruvian man, 219

Walden (Thoreau), 17, 36, 37, 120,
    125, 264
Walker, Lester, 22, 23–24
walls:
  abstract rendering of, 63–64, 97
  and bookshelves, 93, 299
  and corner posts, 89–90
  fin, 93
  glass, 248–57
  height of, 227–28
  load-bearing function of, 250
  memory in, 78
  ninety-degree, 202
  nonexistent, 73
  porches framed by, 264
  thick, 78, 89, 93–94, 97, 277–78
Walpole, Horace, 33
water, and chi, 45–46, 47
white ash, 281–84, 293
Wilson, E. O., 49
windows, 223–66
  aspect ratio of, 254
  building of, 239–45
  and capillary action, 239, 243
  divided-light, 245–46
  and "eight-one," 227–28, 231
  glazing of, 242, 247–53, 258
  installation of, 258–59
  in-swinging, 227, 231–39
  and landscape, 236, 247, 248, 252,
    254–56
  as light source, 75, 77, 246, 248, 262
  muntins on, 245–53, 256
  operation of, 262–63
  peak, 257–58, 259, 262, 270
  people drawn to, 75, 76–77
  perspective from, 10, 12–13,
    27–28, 33, 246, 260–61, 263–65
  picture, 251, 252, 254–56
  on the self, 23
  and space, 236, 249
  and transparency, 246–57, 263–66
  trim, 289–90
  visor over, 94, 95, 287
  and weather, 246

wood:
  finished, 291–93
  for interior space, 281
  lumber as abstraction, 133, 134–35
  vs. steel, 137
  for writing desk, 279–84
wood duck house, 205–7
woodwork, *see* carpentry
Woolf, Virginia, 7–8, 21
words, 53–71, 265
  and architecture, 67–70, 74–78,
    187, 215
  and design process, 57–60
  information overload, 53–54
  reading, 54–56, 70
  reading vs. doing, 56–57, 71
Wright, Frank Lloyd, 105–6, 213,
    273
  centrifugal houses of, 20–21
  Fallingwater by, 102, 181, 201*n*
  and First Shelter, 87
  and Golden Section, 79
  as poet of American ground, 101–2,
    104, 106, 108
  and roofs, 73, 177, 201, 236
  on trees, 135

writing desk, 278–87
  evolution of, 294
  preparation of, 284–86
  shape of, 285–86
  wood for, 279–84
writing hut:
  build it yourself, 5, 21–29
  daydreams about, 14–15
  design of, 90–98
  drawing of, 71–90
  entrance to, 72–73
  as eye-catcher, 34–35
  foundation of, *see* footings
  frame of, *see* framing
  genesis of idea for, 9, 10, 12–14
  lighting of, 297–301
  mental image of, 57–59
  precise angle of, 111
  and primitive hut image, 86–88, 95,
    96, 219
  purpose of, 42
  roof of, *see* roof
  site of, *see* site
  skeleton of, 93
  windows of, *see* windows
  words and, 53–71

This Is Your Mind on Plants

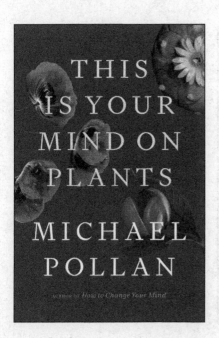

Of all the things humans rely on plants for, surely the most curious is our use of them to change consciousness. In *This Is Your Mind on Plants*, Michael Pollan dives deep into three plant drugs—opium, caffeine, and mescaline—in a radical challenge to how we think about drugs. In this unique blend of history, science, and memoir, as well as participatory journalism, Pollan examines and experiences these plants from several very different angles and contexts, and shines a fresh light on a subject that is all too often treated reductively.

"Expert storytelling . . . [Pollan] masterfully elevates a series of big questions about drugs, plants, and humans that are likely to leave readers thinking in new ways." —*The New York Times Book Review*

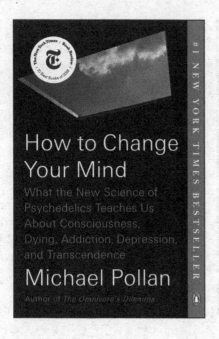

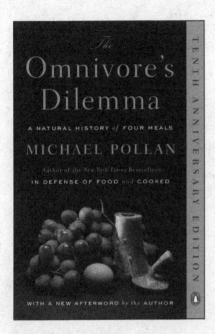
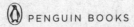

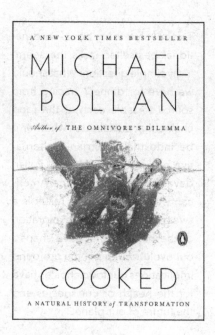
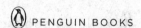